T0223009

Conversations about the NHS

As the National Health Service celebrates 75 years, this book reflects not only on its successes but also on its challenges. Society, medicine and technology have all changed considerably since its founding in 1948 so what can, and should, the NHS do to adapt to remain fit for purpose?

This thought-provoking book is made up of interviews with healthcare leaders, policymakers and practitioners, journalists and patient representatives. Book ended with chapters linking the interviews with the history and the future of the NHS, the book addresses questions such as:

- What are the NHS's strengths and weaknesses?
- How could the NHS be adapted and how should it be set up if founded today?
- How should the NHS recognise the relationship between physical health, mental health, social care and public health?
- How should the NHS be funded?
- How do we understand the social contract between patients, medical and allied professions and the government?
- How can we manage workforce development?
- How should the NHS address issues around social justice and equity of access?

Timely and important, this book promotes debate and critique around key issues in managing healthcare. Relevant to all those working in the NHS, it is also a valuable contribution for healthcare professionals undertaking further study on management and leadership.

All royalties from this book are being donated to The Patients Association.

Dinesh Bhugra is Emeritus Professor of Mental Health and Cultural Diversity, King's College London, UK. Past-President Royal College of Psychiatrists (2008–2011), Past-President World Psychiatric Association (2014–2017), Past-President British Medical Association (2018–2019).

Conversations about the NHS

Dinesh Bhugra

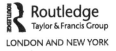

Routledge
Taylor & Francis Group

LONDON AND NEW YORK

Cover image: Jaswant Guzder

First published 2024
by Routledge
4 Park Square, Milton Park, Abingdon, Oxon OX14 4RN

and by Routledge
605 Third Avenue, New York, NY 10158

Routledge is an imprint of the Taylor & Francis Group, an Informa business

© 2023 Dinesh Bhugra

British Library Cataloguing-in-Publication Data
A catalogue record for this book is available from the British Library

Library of Congress Cataloging-in-Publication Data
Names: Bhugra, Dinesh, author.
Title: Conversations about the NHS / Dinesh Bhugra.
Description: Abingdon, Oxon ; New York, NY : Routledge, 2023. |
Includes bibliographical references and index.
Identifiers: LCCN 2023005238
Subjects: LCSH: Great Britain. National Health Service—Public opinion. |
National health services—Great Britain—Public opinion. | Physicians—
Great Britain—Interviews. | Politicians—Great Britain—Interviews. |
Patients—Great Britain—Interviews.
Classification: LCC RA412.5.G7 B57 2023 | DDC 362.10941—dc23/
eng/20230420
LC record available at https://lccn.loc.gov/2023005238

ISBN: 978-1-032-46541-8 (hbk)
ISBN: 978-1-032-46540-1 (pbk)
ISBN: 978-1-003-38218-8 (ebk)

DOI: 10.4324/9781003382188

Typeset in Sabon
by codeMantra

Dedicated to all those who work in the NHS, use it on a daily basis and those who support it.

Contents

Preface

The National Health Service (NHS) came into being on 5 July 1948 and can be seen as one of the proudest achievements of the welfare state and coming together of ideas of universal healthcare irrespective of the ability to pay. From cradle to grave and from physical to mental health and everything else in between, NHS has indeed been a victim of its own success. The expected age of living has increased and also ever increasing number of people are living with multiple complex comorbid conditions. In the 75 years since its inception, the healthcare delivered has changed a great deal. Who would have predicted the use of robots for surgery and telehealth for clinical consultations? Three generations later feelings of gratitude at free healthcare have given way to changed expectations and suitable engagement with patients at an equal level: 'no decision about me without me'. Workforce has changed with a majority of medical students and doctors to be female and generational expectations of proper work-life balance.

The idea for this book emerged not only to celebrate 75 years of the NHS but also to take stock of where we are and where we go but most importantly how do we get there.

As this book goes to press, the country is faced with multiple crises – cost of living, inflation, energy problems and struggles in healthcare system. For the first time in its history, the Royal College of Nursing voted to go on strike and duly did. Ambulance staff and paramedics as well as junior doctors are in line to go on strike. As a result of the pandemic, the waiting lists for elective treatments have grown.

During the Covid pandemic, healthcare workers were being applauded every Thursday evening with clapping and banging of pots and pans and yet the wellbeing of the very same healthcare workers and the stress and pressure they were under did not seem to appear on the political agenda. Pressure on general practitioners was certainly identified, but the blame was placed at their door not recognising the resources needed. The staff vacancy rates among doctors and nurses are unprecedented and yet the demand keeps increasing. Telehealth took a massive leap but pressure on beds, inability to discharge patients who were ready to be discharged and human cost of the pandemic added further stress to already stretched services.

The question arises: if the NHS did not exist and we were starting with a blank sheet of paper would we design it in the same way bearing in mind the medical advances and cross-generational expectations and characteristics? A major tragedy globally has been that health has been seen in a silo as if other factors do not affect it. For decades, if not longer, we have known that social factors affect health, but recently we have come to recognise the importance of geopolitical factors and how these influence social determinants. Cultural, geographical, biological, economic, political and commercial determinants influence health and healthcare and yet education, employment, housing and justice are all considered as if they do not have any impact on the health and wellbeing of individuals. As a result, tragically for ever we are patching people up rather than creating a healthy population. Furthermore, although the UK was a major leader in understanding and stating the role of public health (also known as preventive and social medicine in many countries), not enough attention has been paid to it and it has been isolated by being pushed into local councils who have been deprived of funds in the times of austerity. Separation of public health, physical and mental health and health and social care has compounded the challenges facing the NHS at the present time. This has had horrendous consequences on policy as was evident from the government response to the pandemic.

This book presents transcripts of interviews with a range of people from the past-President of the Royal College of Physicians of London, immediate past-chair of the BMA Council, past chairs of Junior Doctors Committee of the BMA, editor of the Lancet, a Conservative MP, a columnist for the Daily Mail, four members of the House of Lords and the Chair of the Patients Association and its CEO. I am most grateful to all of them for giving their time and expressing their views freely. It is inevitable that when presenting these views in a written format, the passion may not come across but all the interviews were passionate. Every person expressed their views with clarity, and not only their views were well thought-out but they also saw the perilous state of the NHS and had innovative solutions. They were all positive that NHS must survive and prosper even though there were some variations in the process.

I am grateful to Grace McInnes, Amy Johnson and Sarah Rae and their team at Routledge to take the ball and run with it. This project would not have been possible without their unstinting support. Thanks to Martin Deahl and Bex Couper for their help. As always Michael Thacker has been a stalwart in his support, thanks are simply not enough to express my gratitude. Thanks are due to University of Cagliari and Professor Mauro Carta for their support.

Dinesh Bhugra, London
April, 2023

1 Introduction

The NHS: Past and Present

Introduction

National Health Service (NHS) of the United Kingdom has variously been described as being closest to a religion the British have, envy of the world and many other things. It is indeed held with almost religious reverence but also it raises atheistic views. Not a single day goes by when the newspapers are not reporting problems, pressures it is under, resulting low morale and endless policy changes. At the same time almost every day there are reports of new breakthroughs and therapeutic advances. The clapping every week during the pandemic to convey thanks to health workers did not appear out of the blue. The population as a whole recognised the pressures the NHS and its workers were under. Many sick people deliberately stayed away from seeking help. In addition, on a regular basis, newspapers and the media also regularly report new conditions. In lots of ways, the NHS has been a victim of its own success. The average life expectancy of the population has increased by 11 years as has the number of staff and the expenditure per capita.

As we approach its 75th birthday, it is helpful to look at the NHS with a fresh pair of eyes for a number of reasons. The society is not the same as it was in 1948. The attitudes across generations are very different. From a healthcare and social care perspective, people are living longer and doing so with multiple complex long-term conditions. The societal expectations of medicine and healthcare have changed too. Patients in clinical settings want equal partnerships in making any clinical decisions. Often patients present to the services with printouts from the internet asking for specific medications or interventions. In addition, the younger generations have different attitudes to work-life balance, thus adding pressure to workforce levels.

In this chapter, the factors influencing the development and its existence are looked at in some length. This chapter does not aim to provide a full or extensive history of the NHS. There are excellent volumes available on that, some of which are listed at the end of this chapter. For a

DOI: 10.4324/9781003382188-1

number of reasons in this volume, the focus remains on the NHS in England. There are differences across nations, for example, Scotland has integrated social and healthcare which is still missing in England.

Healthcare before the NHS

The NHS as a national service emerged in the aftermath of the Second World War. Until then, the government had very little role to play in healthcare as is the case in a large number of countries around the globe. In many countries, very often there is a mix of private and public healthcare, and often poor people are treated in the public sector with a limited number of drugs, beds, etc. In that respect, the NHS is an astonishing revelation as it is free to access at the point of need for the rich and the poor alike and providing treatment from hernia repairs to heart transplants. The impact of this access is not hard to understand.

In the United Kingdom, until the middle of the 19th century, the government had virtually no role to play in the control of the medical profession for standards or education. Medical Royal Colleges in different disciplines were the bodies which set standards (after a fashion) for education and clinical practice. As different medical specialties emerged and developed, these bodies became more prominent with emergence of various Royal Colleges and Faculties. In earlier periods, the number of doctors practising in London were much larger than those practising elsewhere in the country. London teaching hospitals were much sought after for learning as well as clinical practice.

For the first time in 1834, Poor Law was passed which gave a nod to the fact that governments had a degree of responsibility to look after its population's health. Parish medical officers were made responsible for the care of the health of poor people in specific geographical areas which also had parish workhouses which had sick wards so that those who needed care could be treated (Levitt 1976). Those who were able to pass a means test would get free treatment. In 1848, the Public Health Act established statutory powers that gave a local medical officer of health the responsibility to deliver population health. Subsequently, they were also given a degree of responsibility for providing healthcare in parishes. These responsibilities gradually expanded to include control over school health, district nursing and midwifery services and control of infectious diseases as well as over various environmental hazards. These were a result of local acts from places like London and Liverpool to manage and control infectious diseases. The General Medical Council was established in 1858 to self-regulate doctors and their basic qualifications, and a register of qualified medical practitioners was set up. Stacey (1988) discusses important changes in the mode of healthcare delivery as well as the organisation of the medical profession in the first half of the 20th century. Medical practitioners had gathered a degree of prestige and status, and with the spread of the British Empire, the practice of allopathic medicine was also exported along with colonisation. Consequently, in places like India, the local Ayurvedic healthcare system suffered dramatically. Many institutions teaching Ayurvedic medicine were closed down.

Although medical advances, investigations and study were beginning to give healthcare a more scientific basis, inevitably the reach of medicine in geographical areas remained patchy as medical practitioners continued to stay and practise in cities rather than towns or villages.

In 1911, the National Health Insurance Act was passed which gave workers who fell ill a degree of protection. It meant that the employers, individuals and the state made compulsory contributions and in many ways was the actual precursor of the NHS. At that point in time, this was applicable only to general practitioner (GP) care and individuals from the working classes. The Act did not include hospital care, and the middle and upper classes were seen as being able to afford their own care and were not included. It also did not include workers' families, thereby creating gender, age and disability discrimination (Navarro 1978, Stacey 1988). At that point, although GPs were perhaps the most included, they were also least contented and most vociferous which continued to be the case when the NHS was established in 1948. It was noted that as the GPs were unable to choose their patients and were 'controlled' by a committee of working men "... not a pleasant matter for an educated gentleman to serve under" (BMJ 1875, p 484).

Prior to the 1911 Act, very few working-class individuals could afford GP care through membership of friendly societies, etc. The 1911 Act immediately covered 15 million people, and this figure had risen to half the population (which was about 24 million) by the mid-1940s. The scheme was noted to be inefficient as local insurance committees (precursor of family practitioner committees) as well as approved societies (private insurance companies, friendly societies and trade unions which related to specific occupations and/or locations) controlled access to healthcare services. The failure of these societies was due to complex reasons both financial and administrative. The contributions inevitably changed with earnings. During the latter part of the 19th century and subsequently, healthcare moved from home to hospitals which created an increasing differentiation between specialists and generalists creating a setting of status and tribalism. Honigsbaum (1979) noted that the increasing influence of hospitals created the differentiation under the 1911 Act. Furthermore, this also led to development of a hierarchy not only of the specialties but also that of specialist practitioners. There were approximately 2,800 hospitals (of which 1,000 were voluntary) at the time of the establishment of the NHS. These voluntary hospitals included London teaching hospitals which were comparatively well to-do and non-teaching hospitals which were run by local doctors who combined general and hospital practices. Nearly one third of hospitals were run by hospital specialists who made their living through private practice. Medical appointments to these hospitals were influenced by how much money the specialist could generate through their private practice which still appears to be the case for appointment of specialists in some private clinics. On the other hand, voluntary hospitals were often charitable institutions, likely to be funded by endowments and charity appeals. At the same time, municipal hospitals looked after people through the provision of the Poor Law. Many of the hospitals were ill-equipped and had poor physical structures with poor provision of services.

In 1938, the Emergency Medical Service (EMS) was set up in order to manage war casualties. It took up the financial control but not the buildings. EMS divided England and Wales into 12 regions, and each hospital was categorised by its specific function. During this period, several of the voluntary hospitals became second-line hospitals, and salaried specialists were introduced. This had an impact on the negotiation of doctors' salaries when the NHS was established in 1948. The GPs were allowed to be independent businesses.

Jaques (1978) points out that in order to understand the setting up of the NHS, the following objectives must be taken into account while providing services:

a Clinics, school services, education and other services for prevention and detection of disease.
b Physical treatments including surgical and medical interventions and managing physical and psychological illnesses and impairment.
c Psychological treatments for psychological disturbances and related physical symptoms.
d Educational procedures and provisions of aids to enable the physically and mentally handicapped (sic) to use their abilities as fully as possible.

As Burns and Bhugra (1995) note that very often the NHS is used as a political football. This is a regular topic of tensions between the governing party and the opposition, and yet the politicians often ignore those working in it or even using it apart from paying lip service to the institution. As noted earlier, the idea of the NHS can be dated back to 1911. The essence of the NHS is free care at the point of care for anyone who wants and needs it regardless of the ability to pay. The Dawson Report (by Lord Dawson in 1919) recommended that preventative and curative medicine be combined along with correcting hospital inefficiencies by elected regional authorities and general hospitals brought into line with teaching hospitals in order to improve standards of care universally.

Interestingly, the report made no mention of funding though it argued that salaried services are likely to bring about discouraging initiatives and encourage mediocracy and diminish the sense of responsibility. Other reports such as the British Medical Association (BMA) Proposals for a General Medical Service for the Nation suggested that individuals should be able to choose their GPs who will provide a gatekeeping function for access to hospital specialists. It was suggested that this would be funded by extending the National Health Insurance scheme. Regional disparities in healthcare and outcomes were noted by Political and Economic Planning in 1937. This report identified healthcare as disorganised and suggested that the services needed better coordination.

The Five Giants

Sir William Beveridge in 1942 produced his report on social services and allied services. He saw five giants (want, disease, ignorance, squalor and idleness) as standing in the way of social progress. Eighty years on, none of these giants have been truly slain. There is still want particularly now as the cost of living crisis, inflation and energy crisis begin to bite. Relative poverty levels have increased, and consequently, squalor has not gone. As Timmins (2017) in his magisterial volume notes that the challenge had always been to improve the workings of the welfare state, not how to dismantle it. He reminds us that it is important to know that virtually every day since 1948, the NHS has been said to be in crisis and that in the last 75 years, the morale within it has never been lower. Timmins also reminds us that in the history of the NHS, there was no golden age irrespective of who was in power (p 3) although many politicians often claim to do so. One theme which repeatedly emerged according to Timmins (p 5) is the law of unintended consequences that decisions taken for the best of motives (these so-called repeated reforms, see below) will often go awry.

Beveridge in his paper, Heads of a Scheme in 1941, linked NHS, social security, children's allowances and employment. Bringing together of EMSs, cottage hospitals, teaching hospitals and poorhouses was a major task which needed a lot of political skill and negotiations. Tudor-Hart (1988) describes the state of cottage hospitals where GPs often performed surgery themselves. Timmins (2017, p 102) points out that the NHS is seen as the biggest achievement of the Labour government even though they did achieve other successes.

The tensions between various types of hospitals along with a perception of suspicion never truly went away and to some degree continue even today. The shift to rational control of health services from local control was not universally welcomed, but it occurred nevertheless. The White Paper, A National Health Service, was issued in February

1944 (Timmins 2017, p 111). It was clear that everybody irrespective of means, age, set or occupation shall have an equal opportunity to benefit from the most up-to-date medical and allied services available. The allied services are an interesting aspect in this regard. It could be interpreted that these did not include social care. However, it was clear that services would be available free of charge. These will also be comprehensive and promote good health rather than only the treatment of poor health. Funded by tax and bringing together hospitals and GPs, the service was going to be comprehensive. Working with the presidents of three Royal Colleges – that of Surgeons, Physicians and Obstetricians and Gynaecologists – an agreement was reached for consultants to be awarded merit awards for exemplary clinical work to be judged by their peers and be encouraged to move to various centres around the country. Thus, all the hospitals were brought into government control and nationalised. Thereafter, the GPs were offered a basic salary and niceties. The only condition was to discourage GPs to move into over-doctored areas. Interestingly, Timmins points out that proposals for GPs had been previously put forward by the BMA's own Medical Planning Committee (p 118). Finally, negotiations with the BMA led to the launch of the NHS on 5 July1948. However, Timmins (2017, p 128) notes that "the war over the NHS was to leave the Labour Party deeply suspicious of the BMA for the next 35 years but' it also damaged the standing of the Conservative Party …".

The government plans to move consultants around the country led to deskilling of some GPs as they (as noted above) had previously carried out surgery and anaesthesia and practised as physicians as well. In addition, it would appear that they became more supplicants to the specialists (Timmins 2017, p 129). This also led to a fragmentation of services. Thus, various fragments had different management structures leading to a further sense of tribalism and a divorce between general practice and hospital care. Some of the services were local and others national, and there were additional tensions related to local services as well as special health authorities which created further layers not only of bureaucracy but also a sense of competition, status and tribalism. These changes are said to have led to a fall in the status of the GPs (Timmins 2017, p 129). Pharmacy, ophthalmic and dental services were run by different authorities from hospital or local authority. Along with the arrival of the NHS, social security benefits and welfare state had arrived too.

Early journey of the NHS was not smooth, but the public and patients were grateful that they did not have to pay for healthcare directly and that they did not have to worry if they could not afford to pay. The subsequent path has also been less than smooth for a number of reasons. From increasing demand, expensive investigations and interventions to continual political interference often on ideological grounds have meant that the NHS appears to lurch from crisis to crisis.

Reforms, Re-forms, Re-Re-Reforms

Almost soon after its setting up, there was recognition that reorganisation was needed. Recognising that the demand for health was going to be unlimited, the aphorism 'infinite Demand, finite Resources' was born. A committee was set up to look at the cost of the NHS, chaired by the Cambridge economist C. W. Gillebaud who concluded that the service was not wasteful and it did not require any further reorganisation. Ten years later, the Porritt committee reported that general practice hospital services and community services needed to be unified. Inequalities in funding across geographical regions and across medical specialties continue to persist to date. Klein (1989) noted that the NHS is as much a product of messy compromises as of impaired vision, and the saga continues. There are pockets of excellence and swathes of barely managing services.

The challenges are financial, workforce, lack of planning in the long term as well as politics both with a capital P and a small p. Almost since its inception, the NHS has been beset with 'reforms' often at the behest of politicians. In 1968, there were proposals to integrate services under 50 area boards, but this did not come to fruition. Another Green Paper in 1968 recommended bringing together regional councils, area health authorities and district committees but was abandoned. Following the NHS (Reorganisation) Act of 1973, a year later coinciding with the reorganisation of local government and family practitioner committees were set up. Forsyth (1982) provided a detailed analysis of the political and practical ramifications of the relationship between national and local governments. Furthermore, Draper et al. (1976) offer an overview of the impact of 1974 reorganisation. Since the Griffith Report (1984) commissioned by Mrs Thatcher, the expansion of management in the NHS has continued apace.

The challenges to the NHS continue and are likely to continue further until and unless long-term solutions are found. The chaos in the recent decades has reflected continuing political interference and increasing demand and changed public expectations. There are further specific issues related to the recent pandemic. The breezy slogans that were put out focused on saving the NHS meant that the focus and pressures on the service intensified.

A broad list of some of the changes in the NHS since 1974 is illustrated in Table 1.1.

There is evidence that the introduction of NICE to measure success and value of interventions helped to contain costs and educate the

Table 1.1 Some of the 'reforms' in the last 40 years

1	1982: The Korner report
2	1982: Abolition of NHS area health boards
3	1983: Management budgeting
4	1984: Griffiths report
5	1987: Achieving a balance
6	1988: NHS review
7	1989: Working for patients report
8	1990: NHS and Community Care Act
9	1991: Postgraduate education
10	1991: Trust hospitals
11	1993: Managing the new NHS
12	1997: The new NHS published fundholding eliminated
13	1998: Introduction of clinical governance
14	2000: The NHS plan
15	2001: Primary care trusts set up
16	2002: Wanless report
17	2003: Foundation hospitals
18	2008: Darzi review
19	2009: NHS constitution
20	2010: Liberating the NHS
21	2012: Health and Social Care Act
22	2014: Five-year forward view
23	2016: NHS improvement sustainability and transformation plan
24	2019: Long-term plan
25	2022: Healthcare Act integrated care systems

public and professionals. Roughly at the same time, the chaos caused by Modernising Medical Careers where trainee doctors had to reapply for their posts continues to reverberate to this day. As will become obvious in some of the interviews, the medical profession too has to carry some of the responsibility for potential problems. With the establishment of the Health Education England (HEE), a shared learning programme was envisaged, but this remained properly unfilled. The proposals for 2012 Act caused such an outrage among the profession that the then prime minister paused the reforms. One of the major challenges is that with each reform comes the costs. Mayor (2017) reported that changes due to 2012 reorganisation failed to deliver. Alderslade (1995) describes politics in essence a mechanism for deciding how all those within society with their various aspirations and intentions will live together in some sort of harmony which requires sharing of resources in an appropriate manner. This view is at the core of the social contract between individuals seeking and needing healthcare and professionals on the one hand – a two-way implicit or possibly explicit contract (in private settings) and with the government or the funding bodies such as insurance companies or private providers on the other hand.

Targets set by various governments have been both good and bad. These have, on the one hand, emphasised the advantages so that patients do not wait too long, on the other hand, in many settings, these targets are either ditched or used economically. It is difficult to meet targets, no matter how realistic these are if the healthcare professionals are not available to deliver these.

As countries come out of the pandemic, there are intense pressures on services. Patient demand is high, and in the absence of proper social care, patients are waiting to be discharged from hospitals. Health is determined politically, socially, commercially and culturally, and there are geographic variations too. There is no doubt that the NHS does not have enough beds, doctors, nurses and other staff but also not enough capacity for investigation facilities like MRI scanners which puts additional pressure on staff who are still around.

Conclusions

From this necessarily brief overview, it is clear that the NHS changed the health of the nation in lots of better ways. With those changes came an increase in life expectancy and consequently living with complex co-morbidities. The silo existence of physical and mental health, public health and physical and mental health and health and social care has been damaging to the institution of the NHS and has created difficulties for which patients find difficult to navigate. Development of newer therapeutic interventions has been both expensive and useful. The changes in patient expectations and demands have put additional pressures on healthcare services. Disjunction of public health from health and primary care as gatekeepers has created unexpected consequences which have added further pressures. The challenge is for policymakers and stakeholders to realise and recognise these pressures and put strategies in place now so that the NHS survives both as a principle and as an institution.

Further Recent Sources Especially Related to the Pandemic

www.nhshistory.net

Ashcroft M, Oakeshott I (2022): *Life support: the state of the NHS in an age of pandemics*. London: Biteback

Clarke R (2022): *Breathtaking: inside the NHS in a time of the pandemic*. London: Little Brown.

Haslam D (2022): *Side effects: how our healthcare lost its way and how we fix it*. London: Atlantic Books.

Hennessy P (2022): *A Duty of Care: Britain before and after covid*. London: Allen Lane

Hunt J (2022): *Zero: eliminating unnecessary deaths in a post-pandemic world.* London: Swift Press

References

Alderslade R (1995): The politics, funding and resources of the National Health Service. In D Bhugra & A Burns (eds): *Management for psychiatrists.* 2nd ed. London: Gaskell, pp 18–32

BMJ (1875): Provident institutions and hospitals II: outpatients reforms. *BMJ* 1(745), 483–484

Burns A & Bhugra D (1995): History and structure of the NHS. In D Bhugra & A Burns (eds): *Management for psychiatrists.* 2nd ed. London: Gaskell, pp 3–17

Draper P, Grenholm G, & Best G (1976): The organisation of healthcare: a critical view of the 1974 reorganization of the NHS. In D Tuckett (ed): *An introduction to medical sociology.* London: Tavistock, pp 254–290

Forsyth G (1982): Evolution of the NHS. In D Allen & D Grimes (eds): *Management for Clinicians.* London: Pitman, pp 18–35

Honigsbaum F (1979): *The division in British Medicine: a history of separation of general practice from health care. 1911–1968.* London Routledge Kegan & Paul

Jaques E (1978): *Health service.* London: Heinemann

Klein R (1989): *The politics of the NHS.* London: Longman

Levitt R (1976): *The reorganised NHS.* London: Croom Helm

Mayor S (2017): Major 2012 NHS reforms failed to deliver on promises *BMJ* 359, j5253

Navarro V (1978): *Class struggle, the state and medicine: an historical and contemporary analysis of the medical sector in Great Britain.* London: Martin Robertson

Stacey M (1988): *The sociology of health and healing* London: Unwin Hyman

Timmins N (2017): *The five giants: a biography of the welfare state.* 3rd ed. London: William Collins

Tudor-Hart J (1988): *A new kind of doctor.* London: Merlin Press cited in N Timmins, p 105

2   Lord John Alderdice

Lord John Alderdice is a psychiatrist and medical psychotherapist by profession and a Liberal Democrat peer. As Leader of the Alliance Party of Northern Ireland, he played a significant role in the negotiation of the 1998 Good Friday Agreement and was the first Speaker of the new Northern Ireland Assembly. He has been President of Liberal International, the global network of more than 100 liberal political parties (now Presidente D'Honneur). He is a Senior Research Fellow at Harris Manchester College, Executive Chairman of the Changing Character of War Centre at Pembroke College and has research affiliations with the Department of Politics and International Relations and the School of Anthropology and Museum Ethnography in Oxford. He has established and chairs The Concord Foundation through which he works on his areas of special interest which are the individual and group psychology of terrorism and violent political conflict, the psychology of religious experience and fundamentalism, and the study of relations between groups of indigenous people and settler communities.

Interview

I: Thanks very much for taking the time, really appreciate it. As you know it is the 75th anniversary of the NHS this year so the aim of conversations is to look ahead at what needs changing and what remains the same. I am particularly interested in your views both as a policymaker and as a clinician, but also a Northern Irish perspective. So, if we start with what you see as the problems with the NHS at present and potential solutions and your vision of the future of the NHS.

JA: The idea of doing it as a kind of conversation is very appealing to me. I guess if I start with the part that is almost most distant – that period of time when I was working in the NHS as a consultant psychiatrist in psychotherapy. During that period, I was always working part time for two reasons: firstly, the type of psychiatry that

DOI: 10.4324/9781003382188-2

I was interested in practising was psychotherapy – primarily psychoanalytic psychotherapy, but other kinds of psychotherapy such as family therapy, group therapy and various arts therapies were also of interest to me. The health service itself didn't really provide much option for doing that. As a junior doctor, moving around every 6 months or every 12 months, really was not much use in getting experience in psychotherapy when you have to take the patients on for quite a lengthy period of time. I actually started seeing some patients privately in the evenings when I was a junior doctor. Some members of staff approached me to see their relatives, so I started doing that. There was also another dimension, which was my wish to apply my psychological ideas in politics. I wondered why, if individual people did self-damaging things and we deal with that, when a whole community was behaving in a self-damaging way, why we could not think about doing something about that too. How do we extend those psychological skills? Both in practical terms and intellectually, I've worked for much of my life to try to understand and address that question. I wanted to be fair to the health service and realised that I could not really do those kinds of things and still work full-time in the NHS. Interestingly, things actually worked out very well for me. I was the first and only trainee psychiatrist in psychotherapy in Ireland at that time, and when I finished my training and applied for a job as a consultant psychiatrist in psychotherapy the NHS employers only had money for a part-time job and that suited me fine. I set up a small centre for psychotherapy in Belfast and for some time I could just see things improving a little bit each year. We never had enough money, we never had enough staff, and we were never able to deal with all the people that needed to be seen, so we were very careful about how much we advertised the service because we knew that resources were limited, and we would just get beaten over the head for having large waiting lists. Many patients were from the greater Belfast area, where some GPs were very keen to refer, and others were not. There were other challenges in addition to not having enough therapists. Working with children which could create very difficult situations with childcare hearings and so on. We were fortunate to have some really good people – young trainee psychiatrists, and particularly psychiatric nurses, who had experience of working with really quite disturbed people out in the community. They had a degree of confidence in being able to manage quite disturbed personalities and indeed psychotic patients in the community. They were sensible about it. I found that actually psychiatric nurses were generally excellent, as were some occupational therapists, particularly people who had training in art therapy or music therapy. We developed training courses, including a master's degree course in psychotherapy through the medical faculty at Queen's University. It was going quiet for a number of years. However, in later periods in my career there was more pressure, more difficulty and far less opportunity to develop and innovate. With the arrival of cognitive behaviour therapy, more people learnt the techniques, which was good, but in their enthusiasm, they energetically advertised services, and that was against my advice. As I predicted they got huge waiting lists, and the staff couldn't cope with it. It was fine to have ambitions for the kind of service you would like to provide, but increasing demands contributed to increased pressures from the public and on the healthcare workers. Resources were limited and increasing demands just increased pressures. Opportunities for training were also limited which itself led to further pressure and difficulties. This led to my small service having to take on many of the patients on their waiting lists.

Not long after that I decided to retire from clinical practice to devote more of my time to politics. I had been in the House of Lords as a member of the Liberal Democrat peers since 1996. And in 2010, I was appointed the health spokesman in the Lords for the Liberal Democrats. After the May 2010 election, there was a Conservative/Liberal Democrat coalition government, and I was elected Convenor of the Liberal Democrats – the chair of the backbench Lib Dems. I was also co-chair with John Pugh MP of the Lib Dem Health Group, and I spent a lot of time on the development of the Health and Social Care Bill. There was a sense that the managerial approach, that had been going on for some decades, with professional managers, who came into the NHS with a good business sense from all sorts of backgrounds, really wasn't working at all. It wasn't working for a very fundamental reason – because it is not the same thing dealing with healthcare. If you are running a business and there is something that does not produce a profit, you stop doing it and change. You acknowledge that service does not sell or is not popular and you change the business. But you can't turn to people with cystic fibrosis and say, "You are not really getting better so we will not bother treating people like you because it doesn't pay". That is not what the healthcare system is about. The business ethos and the business manager approach simply isn't an appropriate approach for an NHS. What I and other colleagues were keen to do with this legislative opportunity was to have clinicians, who had some understanding of what a health service was about, play more of a role in management. My feeling was that the doctors in general had become institutionalised in the health service. They should not be able to keep saying that this is nothing to do with them and then continue to complain. Our thinking was that they must take responsibility for resources and sensible spending. We took the view that we cannot continue to demand more and more resources without having to take any responsibility for managing them. There was a great struggle in the coalition government about this, between those of us who felt that it was important for clinicians to be involved in the managerial decisions and to encourage responsibility for deciding what kind of care there should be, and indeed for prioritising and maybe even rationing, not a word that people wanted to use at all, but really, it was essential. In the end, it did not work because there were a number of key colleagues in my own party and elsewhere who, having come up through the old NHS way of providing healthcare, wanted to continue in the same way. The key one was Shirley Williams who had been a Labour Government Minister. She has been one of the Gang of Four who left Labour and created the SDP and then merged with the Liberal Democrats. She was a lovely grandmotherly figure who was a great speaker. Shirley was a national icon, and you could not confront her. When she linked herself up with the health service issue and opposed your proposals for other ways of working, it wasn't possible to deliver it. The Lib Dem leader, Nick Clegg, actually did try for a little while, but he discovered that he was on what we would call 'a hiding to nothing'. Shirley was able to appeal to people's wish that whatever healthcare they wanted – not even needed but wanted – should be available to them free at the point of delivery. I could see that this was desirable, but it is not deliverable because there is an endless demand for all sorts of care. There is just no end to this increasing demand. We were inventing new medications and new approaches to treatment, and the costs were increasing endlessly. We also have an increasingly elderly population, and we were bringing people in from outside the country to look after them, which was becoming increasingly unpopular. People did not want large-scale immigration. And yet the health service was depending, for example, on excellent people from the Philippines. There were marvellous nurses and doctors from elsewhere who people loved, but if you said that they were coming as immigrants, people did not want that. The effort to make the changes was not getting anywhere because we couldn't deliver it politically. As a result, I withdrew from that portfolio and increasingly involved myself with the other major area of my interest, which was dealing with an intractable violent political conflict and other specific issues such as the regulation of psychotherapy, which still remains a concern of mine, and I keep coming back to it. However, the problems that I had seen in the management of the NHS at that stage and tried to do something about seem to me have simply got worse.

Another area of concern was social care. I remember bringing Andrew Dilnot in to meet my parliamentary colleagues and he produced and explained his excellent report. We knew what was needed and we tried to persuade colleagues to do it. They went halfway down the road, but when it came to finance and implementation, the agreement fell apart. In response to your very first question about the state of the NHS, at the present time? I could say it in two words – "It's broken". The health service is broken. It doesn't work anymore. People keep on saying that we have the best health service in the world, but we don't. The health service is not serving people properly, and it can't. It is a disaster now for patients and for staff of all kinds and at all levels. I've seen it myself. We have three children and six grandchildren. The care of young mothers going in for obstetric care is a disgrace. Often they are admitted too late and discharged too early, and they end up in all sorts of difficulties. I have seen this in our own family. Young mothers-to-be are not brought in early enough, not looked after properly and then they're pushed out after a day or so even though they have been through a very difficult physical and emotional event. And when they do go back home, they not only have to look after themselves and the baby but also the house and a household. Most of them are unable to call on family because family are at a distance and there are all sorts of pressures. That is only one example of how the NHS is broken, but in all sorts of areas, it is absolutely clear to me that the NHS isn't working.

While the Covid pandemic did show the value of having a National Health Service, it also showed how it was not coping. As it has done in almost every other area, the pandemic exaggerated and exacerbated problems that were already there. In general, it is not that it created entirely new problems, but it made the problems that were already there very much worse. It both exaggerated and exacerbated them, and in my view, it has left health service staff burnt out. They're absolutely exhausted, and many good people are leaving. If you add to Covid the problems that the Treasury has created with the pensions for consultants, we are finding that many key people in the later part of their career, when they are the most experienced and best capable of deciding about services and training the next generation, are disappearing. My wife, who has also retired as an NHS histo- and cyto-pathologist, was a year younger than me in medicine at Queen's University in Belfast. When we go to our medical reunion dinners, we find that most consultants have taken early retirement. This is in contrast with our classmates who went to Canada and are still working. When you ask them, "Why are you still working?" the response is that they enjoy the work and in Canada they can make their own decisions about how to manage things. They do not have people looking over their shoulder all the time stopping them or checking administratively what they are doing like they do here. They have kept on working for much longer. It wasn't that people fell out of love with the clinical aspects of their jobs, but people could not stand the managerial requirements that were being forced on them in the NHS. My wife enjoyed her job but took early retirement because of pressures of administration and management, and she is not alone in this. So, what is the short answer to your question, "What about the health service?" My answer is, "The health service is broken".

You asked about its strengths and weaknesses. Well, it does have strengths. One of its great strengths that was evident during Covid pandemic was its national coverage, so data can be collected nationally, vaccines can be rolled out nationally and tests can be organised nationally. When you look at what happened in the United States, which does not have a national health service, they were quite unable to do these things so effectively. So, that is a big strength. But the weakness is that it is based on an illusion about what can be delivered with a system that is totally dependent on taxation that is central and delivery to everybody of whatever they want, whenever they want it. That's just not possible. I don't think that that can be managed with a health system of the kind that we have, based solely on general taxation with things that are free at the point of delivery for whatever you want, whenever you want it. I just don't think it's possible.

I: I think you raise some very pertinent issues. Having spent 40 years or so in the NHS, I've seen the managerialism. Certainly, in psychiatry, clinicians stayed away from management because they felt they were clinicians primarily and they focused on that. In practice often you got people going into management, many of whom held grudges against doctors, so they took on those roles to 'get even'. If you were redesigning the NHS, what would you do differently, given what you talked about? We know that the demand is increasing with people living longer with multiple complex conditions. New interventions and investigations are expensive. People's expectations have also changed. So how do we bring all that together? It is also about rights and responsibilities of patients but also rights and responsibilities of clinicians. How do we try and have a dialogue? We are certainly not having a dialogue at the moment.

JA: You're completely right. It is very difficult to persuade political colleagues to engage in any sort of dialogue or conversation that goes beyond demands for more money, but it is absolutely essential now.

I hope I'm not being unfair, but I think that within the Conservative government not only is there a recognition of a number of these problems, but a wish to try to do something about them. But it is not doing it in an open or a sensible way. So, for example, when one tries to suggest looking at workforce planning, often the response from politicians is that it is 'not our job'. Of course it is part of their job, but I think part of the reason why it is not being done properly is that there is a push to get more and more non-medically qualified (and therefore less expensive) people to do things that medically qualified people should be doing. As a result, we have a lower number of medical practitioners per head of population than almost any other country in Europe, but nobody wants to speak to it, or address it. Things are going to get worse because experienced doctors, as I was saying earlier on, are leaving. So how can you try to address this?

Well, I think there are some systemic things that are worth considering. I mentioned our experience in Northern Ireland, and one of the things that did happen there – a good thing that came out of the political problems – was the integration of health and social care. It did not address all the problems, but it led to a greater degree of co-operation. There are all sorts of difficulties in health and social care in Northern Ireland, and not least because of the absence of political leadership, and there are other reasons that are very specific to Northern Ireland such as a politically divided society, and disagreements about what people want from the service, but the system of integrated health and social care is a good thing. It seems to me that it is essential for England too. One of the problems that we have had here is Accident and Emergency units being completely blocked, and ambulances unable to do other things but sitting outside the hospital because there are no beds for their patients. Meantime in the hospitals are patients who could be discharged and should no longer be in-patients but instead should be in social care. I think that one contributor to this is that health and social care are operating with different budgets, different managers and different systems – they're not collaborating sufficiently closely. Social care is a local authority responsibility, and the NHS is a national responsibility and neither work very well anymore. There are systemic things that can be done. Again, this was something we wanted to do in the 2011 Health and Social Care Bill. There were some pilot schemes, but it has not developed in the way that it should. That remains for me, one of the important elements of the system that needs to be addressed – the integration of health and social care. We also need to deal with the bureaucracy that was created but which hasn't worked. It was never going to work well because people wouldn't face up to some of the facts honestly. But these issues need to be addressed.

There are other issues too, which I would describe as cultural ones. One of these is the notion that we should simply have a publicly owned and run health service and that anything else is really a bit distasteful. There is a view that any private sector care or community sector care is really a failure to provide the fundamentally 'good thing', which is a national health service, publicly funded, providing for everybody. Anything else is just not good. I think we need to change the culture to say something different. It is not simply about a health system that is only a safety net, but it is about collaboration that people bring to the system through different ways of working partly because we don't have a perfect model anywhere in the world; therefore, having different models within your national system means one can pilot, experiment and see what works better and what doesn't work. In any case, what might work in the Highlands of Scotland might not be the best thing for Central London, so you need to have a diversity of provision since we have different communities with different problems and needs. We do not have one perfect model, and therefore, a degree of experimentation is important and necessary if we are to improve our provision of health and social care. This requires a culture change in the community as a whole to appreciate that diversity of our system is good and not something to turn your nose up at.

The second thing is about responsibility. A problem with the NHS is that it has created a notion that the responsibility for healthcare is a government responsibility. It is not seen as a responsibility of professionals or of patients. As a doctor I need to be responsible in my engagement, not just as a specialist but as someone who addresses the whole patient, the patient in the family, in the community, in the country and in the overall environment. As a doctor, I need to take an interest in and responsibility for as much as I can in all of these areas. The circumstances in which the family is living – poverty and other factors – are important as a doctor and should be part of a doctor's thinking and engagement with the patient.

The patient also plays a role. We cannot say that it is always someone else's fault that the patient is sick. It's not about fault. It's about all of us having to take some degree of responsibility for ourselves and for each other too. I am no great fan of Boris Johnson, but one thing that he said was absolutely right. It was after he was sick with Covid and he said, "The National Health Service is the way that we take responsibility for each other when each other is not well". I think that the notion of how we take responsibility for ourselves and for each other as people and as citizens is important, but it needs a culture change. So, how do we get people to take some more responsibility for their health? This requires money and effort. People need to be prepared to do things. One of the consultants during our training held the view that after the visit to hospital, in that case childbirth, every woman, or every couple, should get a bill on discharge. It doesn't matter how accurate the bill is, but stamped on the bill should be: **Paid by the NHS**. His point was that people need to know there is a cost to this, and somebody somewhere is paying for it. I actually think it needs to go further than that now. For example, in France, the government takes responsibility for 80% of the cost with most people, but you have got to take some responsibility for the rest. I travel quite a lot. On one occasion, I called in to the general practice surgery near my home in Belfast to get some tests done before I set out to travel. There were a couple of older men sitting beside me in the waiting area having a chat with each other. One said to the other, "I didn't see you here last week" and the other said, "No, I really wasn't very well". Coming to the doctor had become part of their social life, more than whether they were well or not. Indeed, if they weren't well, they didn't come. I think we need to change the culture, not just the systems. There needs to be a change of attitudes and I think that may require some modest financial contribution from everybody. People say that will put some people off. Well, yes, that may be so, but could it be that it is because they are not prepared to take responsibility for their own health? Do they feel that somebody else should take responsibility for their healthcare? They take responsibility for purchasing their own food and clothes, why not some contribution to healthcare? There is no easy answer that solves all the problems or addresses every situation. I read a report recently from a group called Radix – a centre-left think tank – who were talking about the need for a hypothecated tax for healthcare so that everybody has to pay, but it is a tax only for healthcare. There are a number of things about that. First of all, if it is a hypothecated tax and people have to pay it, why is it best that it's paid through the tax system? People don't really identify that it's to do with health, whereas if they were paying through some other system or an insurance system or whatever, it would be clear this is what it is for. Secondly, hypothecated tax doesn't seem to work well in the United Kingdom. Let me give you an example. When Paddy Ashdown was leader of the Lib Dems, everybody was talking, not about health but about education. We came up with this proposal for a hypothecated tax – a penny on tax for education. When we did some opinion polling, everybody said that was a great idea; focus groups were positive too and so we started campaigning on 'a penny on the tax for education'. About three days before the election, all the positive sounds turned negative because people began to realise that this was an extra penny on tax, and they didn't want to pay any more tax. Several things came out of that for me. One is that there is a limit to how much one can get people to pay in tax. It is different at different stages, but at the moment, people don't want to pay any more tax. The second thing is hypothecating that tax; while it sounds like a very good idea, it does not make any difference if people are being asked to pay more tax. So, it is actually better to take it at least partly out of the tax system and have it paid for in another way whether that's insurance or something else.

I mentioned Andrew Dilnot earlier. His approach was that there is a maximum amount that people should have to pay for their social care, and at that point, the government should take responsibility for the rest. There were specific arrangements proposed in his report for dealing with those who have disabilities and those who are elderly and so are particularly vulnerable. He put together an excellent report, and people need to take that report out and implement it. Some of the legislation is already in place, but the Treasury keeps saying that it cannot be done. If we did implement it for social care, we would be heading in the right direction. That is not a hypothecated tax, but rather letting people know that they have to pay and also that they know what they are paying for, but that they are not paying over the odds. I don't like the term 'hotel charges', but there is a case for a limited contribution to 'accommodation costs'. That is the kind of approach that I would be wanting to take the next year if I was in a position to try to design the NHS or press for it myself.

I: Very few people know what they're paying for. At the moment, healthcare is just seen as a deep well from which people can keep drawing. Another thing that you highlighted, which I am very much in favour of, is capability to be healthy and a social contract. Capability to be healthy can be seen as a pyramid. At the bottom of the pyramid is the government, which gives you the right information. Above that is the community responsibility; then the family responsibility; and on top is individual responsibility to be capable and be healthy. If you have the right information and you still continue to smoke and you're not accessing smoking cessation services, then maybe there is something that you need to be doing to help yourself. As you say integration of health and social care is absolutely vital, how do you see integration of physical and mental health and public health and physical health? Public health has been hived off into local councils' agenda along with social care, which creates more problems. Of course, there are and should be national standards, but implementation and delivery has to be local – who takes charge of that?

JA: Yes, you are absolutely right. There are a number of things I would say about that. The first is that I agree with the idea of national standards for many, if not all of the things that we do. People may need to be helped at local level to deliver those standards in the context in which they are living. One of the things that was clear to me during the pandemic was that when the government tried to deliver everything at a national level, it was just too much. It was not possible. But when you went down to a local level where people knew where people lived and they knew the requirements in local schools, etc., then these could be delivered. Everybody knew that people were trying to deliver in principle the same kind of tests, the same kind of vaccinations everywhere, but it had to be done in different ways in different places. Public health at a local level is actually very important and consulting with local people about how to deliver it is very important for it to be accepted. There also has to be a public health approach at the national level. There are some things that need to be procured at a national level and national standards are important too, but we ought to be aware of differing attitudes at local levels. One of the people who was very significant in the early days of the development of ideas about of public health in this country was a Glasgow physician called J.L. Halliday. His approach to illness led him to ask these essential questions – why does this person fall ill at this time with this particular kind of problem, and what kind of person is this? Remember we are talking about a public health physician. What he really was saying was, I need to understand why this person falls ill at this point? Is it to do with their family situation? Is it to do with their mental health? Is it to do with the physical situation that they find themselves in? Is it to do with the economic situation? Why do they fall ill this time with this problem and not with another problem? And we also need to consider what kind of person are we dealing with, because that will also give us the answer to a lot of these questions. When you see illness in that way, you have developed a bio-psycho-social model of sickness and health. One of many problems about much of our training and teaching and a lot of our services is that the bio-psycho-social factors are all split off from each other rather than understanding that they are intimately connected; interconnected but not muddled. There is a complexity about us as human beings and our society that is not reducible to linear simplicities. That requires a development of our thinking and our culture and our way of understanding things. We should be able to do this as psychiatrists because we have a medical training, and we have a psychological training, and we should also have an understanding of society. One of the tragedies is that sometimes psychiatrists don't feel that they are 'real' doctors, and so they narrow their approach to one of being only biological psychiatrists, leaving others who address only the psychological side and still others who become social psychiatrists. It all becomes very reductionist. This splitting loses us the tremendous opportunity to help our colleagues in medicine, in sociology, in psychology and even in public policy by bringing all these things together. I think we have a tremendous opportunity as psychiatrists because we have a chance of bringing the biological, psychological, sociological as part of the same phenomenon of being human.

I think that this is part of a larger cultural change that needs to take place. In other work that I do on societal conflict, I find that I benefit by paying more attention to indigenous peoples and first nations and how they try in a traditional way, to see life and society as a whole, of which they are a part. It is a way of thinking about things that I find important, not because they have the answer to everything – obviously they don't – but that notion that we are all a part of something bigger than ourselves. We are not looking down on the environment and being stewards of it, we are part of the environment. It is a different way of thinking about things.

I: You are absolutely spot-on. Mind-body dualism separates out mind and body as if they do not communicate with each other. Other healthcare systems, such as Ayurveda, link mind and body as they affect each other and they are influenced by weather, diet, environment, etc. We may see that as unscientific, but there's something holistic. Another challenge for the NHS is workforce planning. I am sure there have been multiple reports on the subject but as I see it the workforce planning is simply not good enough. Related to that is the role of doctors and nurses. Do you think there is some mileage in doing some part of the training jointly across various disciplines?

JA: I think there can be value in it. But I also think that different professions are different for a reason, and it is not just about what kind of A-levels or O-levels you need to get into the different professions but because they have different sets of attitudes. One of the things that I've noticed, and I mentioned this earlier, is that I found that psychiatric nurses often make excellent psychotherapists. On the other hand, I find that a lot of other nurses, including many who are nursing managers, operate more on the basis of protocols than of professionalism. To my mind, one of the tragedies in medicine is that we have been pushed down the road of protocols rather than professionalism. I believe that is both unhelpful and unhealthy. I think there is something valuable about a doctor who understands the up-to-date way of looking at things but is then able to note that this person in front of him/her has the same symptoms as that of another person, but that they have different underlying pathologies. The danger, in psychiatry in particular, is that if one looks only at symptoms and can tick all the boxes on a protocol, one thinks one understands the problem and there is then a straight line to the treatment. That can be a mistake because people are much more complex than that. Being a good doctor involves dealing with that degree of complexity.

I think there needs to be absolute respect between professionals working together, but I fear that sometimes ends up in a muddled mess. The government then decides that since doctors are more expensive, we do not really need doctors. We can simply get nurses and pharmacists to prescribe all kinds of things. Now there are certain contexts, where that is appropriate. In Tanzania, for example, many years ago, they developed the so-called 'barefoot doctors' who could diagnose and treat ten common diseases in their local area. They knew when it wasn't one of those and then sought help. But we're not living in Tanzania, and we should be able to understand more than that. I have some anxieties about inter-professional education, but my concerns can easily be addressed. When I was training psychodynamic psychotherapists, for example, whether they were doctors, nurses or social workers, they all come along to the same course. I found that their core professions gave them different sets of attitudes and understandings, and so they had different contributions to make whenever they were operating as trainee psychotherapists. So, I am not against joint educational courses, but if it is not done in a thoughtful way, without understanding the specifics of the different professions and respect for their various contributions, it can end up in a mess.

You mentioned the questions of e-learning and telehealth, and this is something that I looked at recently. I was the only medical member of the House of Lords Committee on Covid – a special committee that was set up to look at the likely long-term consequences of the pandemic. We produced a number of reports, and initially, we thought that we would be coming out the other end of Covid before the committee's mandate ended. However, when we finished, we still weren't out the other end, so you must take some of our thoughts with a pinch of salt. One of the things that did become clear to us was that while the pandemic did reveal things that could be done better in telemedicine and online, it also revealed to us the dissatisfaction that many doctors and patients felt about an inappropriate use of online treatments and facilities, especially when people want to see a doctor or nurse in person because they wanted to be seen as a whole person and not just the little bit on the screen. A general practitioner, complained to me that he had not become a doctor to work in a call centre but to engage in person with patients – to see whole patients walking in, walking out, engaging with him and him knowing where they come from. He was in a health centre in the locality which patients knew well and where they had attended his father and grandfather who had been GPs there before him. There are many ways in which online facilities can help, but if we become infatuated with telehealth and think that it can solve all the problems, we simply won't provide a good health service. One of the greatest dangers that I can see is that because people think telemedicine is a cheap way of providing services, they will go for it despite the limitations. We have all seen that with Zoom. Some relationships have bloomed online, but there are some aspects of relational life that you just can't do online.

I: The point that the GP is making is a good one. Maybe we are in a period of transition, so everyone is adjusting to doing medical consultations in different ways. Medical students have told me that they find it difficult to deal with simulation as at the back of their mind they know that this person is not a real patient but is being paid to be so and they are not able to generate empathy. We seem to be blindly going on with it as if this is the Holy Grail and we must follow it, otherwise we'll get lost, and we're not picking up the subtleties and nuances and the pressure that puts people under.

JA: There is another element to it, Dinesh, and it is about relationships. You know, care is fundamentally not about protocols. Care is a relationship between at least two people, and when one forgets that and simply deals with patients according to protocols the notion of relationship is lost.

I: Earlier, you touched upon the rights versus responsibilities of patients. There is also the question of the social contract between medicine and society and vice versa but also both parties have a contract with the government. I wonder if you want to expand on that?

JA: There are a couple of things that I would say about it. The first refers back to what I was saying earlier about this notion of taking responsibility, each of us in our own way. We cannot hand over the responsibility for our lives to somebody else, whether that's the government or a healthcare professional. They can't have 100% of the responsibility, though they may have a significant amount of it. I think the term social contract is itself a bit of a problem because it makes it out to be a legal thing, whereas it is about the relationships that we have with each other. Those relationships involve rights and responsibilities, but they also involve something that is the essence of human nature as individuals and community. I am afraid we have lost some of that and finding our way back to it is really important.

Then, there is a second element of the social contract, in which generations of people entered into an understanding with the government where they agreed to pay their taxes and in return expected the government to be there when they got old and sick. However, this aspect of the social contract also fails to address the complexities. The level of care and treatment now expected is much greater, and if it is felt by the government that they cannot address such changes in the social contract, we may find them forced into radical shifts rather than evolutionary transitions.

Relationships are also important in any such process and that's another thing about the social contract. If we are changing it, as I think we must, where is the 'contract' between current taxpayers and the government. All this has to be managed over a period of time. No matter what we do, it will be a bit bumpy, but we can't forever delay or dismiss the need for change.

I: Thanks very much John, that has been incredibly helpful. Is there anything else that you want to say that we have not covered?

JA: I don't think there's anything more that I would say other than to emphasise the urgency of dealing with the problems. We cannot continue with massive waiting lists and catastrophic collapse in morale amongst healthcare workers. There is an urgency. You and I thought that there was an urgency in 2010 and that's why there was a Health and Social Care Bill. For all the reasons I've mentioned, it hasn't delivered what we wanted, and 12 years on, things are no better, if anything, they are much worse, and we are heading into a virtual collapse in some areas. In truth, we may already be into the early days of that collapse. We have got to deal with the problems, and it needs to be done urgently.

I: Thanks very much, John. Really, really appreciate your time.

3 Lord Nigel Crisp

Lord Nigel Crisp is an independent crossbench member of the House of Lords where he co-chairs the APPG on Global Health. He was Chief Executive of the NHS England and Permanent Secretary of the UK Department of Health from 2000 to 2006. He now works and writes mainly on global health with a focus on Africa. He has published several books on the state of the NHS and also on global health, especially training matters. His current focus is on creating health – promoting the causes of health – developing the health workforce and improving health globally. Lord Crisp is a Senior Fellow at the Institute for Healthcare Improvement, an Honorary Professor at the London School of Hygiene and Tropical Medicine and a Foreign Associate of the US National Academy of Medicine. He was formerly a Distinguished Visiting Fellow at the Harvard School of Public Health and Regent's Lecturer at Berkeley.

Interview

I: Thanks very much for agreeing to be interviewed and making the time. What do you see as the state of the NHS at the present time?

NC: Well, it's difficult to see, as it has got a hill to climb and I suspect this new prime minister, depending on who it is, may make life more difficult and they may be less sympathetic to the NHS. And again, it depends upon who it happens to be because we've got some extraordinary people with very extreme views standing (elections for Conservative Party leadership were going on at the time of this interview). You might see some really damagingly disruptive things. I have my own view about what needs to be done disruptively, but positively, I think.

I: It would be really helpful to hear that as well because it is not only about the problem, but it's also what solutions. And in your book, *24 Hours to Save the NHS*, I think you covered a lot of what I am hoping to talk about today anyway.

DOI: 10.4324/9781003382188-3

NC: I won't repeat much of that because that was about 20th century ideas – it was written in the first decade of this century but addressed reforms that were really all about 20th century ideas. I think in many ways the 21st century is only just starting, and I think life needs to shift radically. If you think of the two biggest problems that are facing health systems globally. Well, there are three actually but let us just start with the first two. The first one is the workforce and health workers. The number of health workers are spread unevenly around the world and this compounded by the poaching of them from different countries. The morale and the epidemic of exhaustion, across health professionals including nurses in a number of countries, is a major issue. This is making the situation extraordinarily unstable. The second thing is that we have not yet worked out in our health systems how to tackle the social determinants of health and the wider determinants of health. And in the report we are publishing tomorrow, we are saying that we have got to tackle these. And the only way to tackle these issues is firstly for a vision for the health system that is about engaging all parts of society in promoting health and creating health and preventing disease. I am very clear that it is about creating health and not just preventing disease through the causes of health and not just the causes of disease. Secondly, within that position, health workers can have a greater role as agents of change and curators of knowledge. By that I mean they are the people who can advise, influence, facilitate, shape, not tell, both at the individual level for dealing with the individual patient and talking to the patient about food or whatever and seeing the patient in the round rather than simply in terms of the body system. However, at another level, they have a role in supporting the community. That includes things like social prescribing, advocacy and as curators of knowledge. The last is really important as we are living in strange times where truth is seen as being relative, isn't it? It is negotiable. It is not absolute. So, who are the people we should turn to? The people we trust most are nurses. And after that, we trust doctors. They have a role about curating, not teaching. As curators of knowledge making knowledge available and accessible to people in ways that they get it. So that is the second part of my vision. The third part of the vision is very obvious that the greatest focus needs to be on services delivered at home or in the community and as locally as possible. Of course, it is important to recognise that there will always be a need for specialist services which will be centralised and needing quick access to them. So if the first issue is human resources, the second issue is what health workers will be doing in the future and the third is local delivery for which technology will play a big role.

Science and technology will change things dramatically in the next 15–20 years. It will shape how people think, about not only the current state and the future, but also about what is possible. And it is really important that we get ready for that. Unfortunately at the present moment there is very little sign that we will. And I think the technology will develop faster than the systems to catch up with it. But those are the three big issues and they affect every health system in low middle income, high income countries and the NHS is just the local example, if I can put it like that. But I think, you know, obviously I'll try and persuade the new Prime Minister of this, but I don't expect to get anywhere. But you know, this is fundamental stuff. It's 21st century health as opposed to the industrial model that we had in the 20th century. And incidentally, the idea of health workers as agents of change and curators of knowledge restores some of the professionalism that has been lost by people in recent years. Protocols and systems tell them what to do and turn them into technicians and create some of the angst that is around about people questioning what their jobs are and thinking what's the point? Changing the role may bring people back into a different set of professional values. I think that will help with morale in that way. We tried in the 20th century to change systems and incentives which worked to an extent. But now we need to get into motivation and away from incentives though they are linked. So that is my manifesto.

I: That is really helpful. Throughout years of our training we are never taught about advocacy for a patient. We just stumble along and learn, while some people are very good, most of us are not. I like your concept of curating because this holding the knowledge and then sharing it and making it possible for people to pick the right messages. You mentioned social determinants and that's where inter-national health comes in, which is about the geo-political determinants, whether war, conflict, famine, migration, etc. affect social determinants at the national level. How do you think that we can try and curate that debate? Because people might say, well, this is not in my hand. I can do nothing about it.

NC: You may not be aware that for the past 10–15 years there has been an interesting course run in Geneva at the Graduate Institute called Health Diplomacy, which is precisely about that area and is precisely how health is going to be part of foreign policy. When we talk about the social determinants of health it is about the social, physical, environmental and political and economic determinants. The political determinants of health are just as important as any others, in some ways more important. I mean, economic is also very important. My most recent book, *Turning the World Upside Down*

Again: Global Health in a Time of Pandemics, Climate Change and Political Turmoil, does pick up on that point. We know that only 3% of world trade goes through Africa. So while Africa is excluded from world trade in that way, it is never going to be able to climb out of poverty. So, there are huge economic factors at play. As you say wars and conflicts are important too and health is affected by all of these. Of course, global institutions like the WHO have a vital role to play although they are partly hamstrung because they rely on contributions from states. But there are plenty of other groups at a global level who could be much more influential. Indeed more people from health backgrounds should be going formally into politics but doing so on the basis of a changed professional education. As you just said, you weren't taught about any of this. And even though you're a psychiatrist now, you had to learn the bones in the foot, didn't you? The whole thing has to shift. And again, in our latest reports and, indeed, in my last book we spelt out a different way of delivering professional education, which people have been working on for some time. It's not my idea but I am reporting this. I think that actually what will happen in health is related to what will happen inside the heads of health professionals. If you see health differently, health will be different. And unfortunately we tend to spend all this time talking about systems. Of course we need systems, but the stuff gets done despite the systems. We hear from clinicians that they sometimes need to bend the system to get their patients what is needed. There is an old fashioned 20th century way of looking at this – the industrial model of health and systems and incentives which is essentially an economic and capitalist framework. And there's a 21st century way of looking at it, which is much more about influence, narrative quality, relationships and professionalism, actually different sorts of professionalism.

I: What do you see as the strengths and weaknesses of the NHS?

NC: Well, all of the above. It has major problems with health workers and the use of technology. It also has major problems with its focus on prevention because it is doing so in a hopelessly bureaucratic fashion. Actually it needs disruption, but a good sort of disruption. My starting point for such a disruption would be a new prime minister coming in and saying that we understand that 80% of a person's health is affected by what happens to them at school, at work, in the family and the community. So we need to launch a whole programme of mobilising society to promote and improve health and create health. There must be an understanding that you create health not simply by preventing individual diseases, but through creating the environment and conditions in which people can be healthy and help others to be so.

I: As you say the NHS needs a bit of disruption and the role of health professionals has to shift and change. Where do we begin? How do we make the NHS fit for purpose?

NC: Well, you begin outside the NHS. You cannot reform the NHS from inside. You can only fiddle. I don't know much about the NHS these days, I'm happy to say, but I see from the papers that, for example, people are creating surgical hubs. Well, great. You know, you get a few more patients seen but it is not strategic. And it's not significant. The starting place has to be outside the NHS. The NHS can't reform itself.

I: The demand keeps increasing and more expensive interventions are coming and more people want those expensive interventions quite rightly, but nobody's prepared to pay for it.

NC: But that's the wrong question, Dinesh. It is phrased in economic language. When did you start talking about supply and demand instead of needs and services? That is what we have done so far. The right question is how do we create a healthy society? Not how do we help the NHS? We are just going to have to patch up the NHS while we get other things right. The reality is that nobody is going to want to pay more.

I: I find it quite interesting that very often people want something but they do not want to or able to take responsibility for their own health.

NC: Well, that's too individually focused. There was a letter in *The Times* today just reminding people that before the war, it was a responsibility for people to have health insurance schemes and to keep themselves healthy. And they could be fined if they didn't keep themselves healthy. But that's all individual focused. There are actually four arenas for improving health. One is individual and nothing I'm saying should detract from that. So if I have a nasty cancer, I want the most specialised technical person. Then there is the community level, which is where you belong, whether you have a community of place or a community of identity or whatever and what happens to you in that. Then there is the society level, which is where you come up against the big economic issues and inequality, etc. And then there is the planetary level. So at all levels including the planetary level, there are different things that we should be doing about health. Any sensible health policy for the future will need to address health across these four arenas, and at each level, it needs to be done in different ways. At the moment, the NHS is still just focused on the individual. Slowly it is trying to move primary care towards communities, but it's doing so in a clunky top-down sort of way. One of your questions is about examples of good practice. There are people advocating at primary care level. A surgery in

Horley is running something called growing health together where part of the time and part of the work is actually spent with people outside in the wider community. There people are doing things which are creating health and growing health together. That is a mini version of what I think we need. We need a massive political drive, but you cannot reform the NHS from inside.

I: The four levels that you mention are exactly the basis of social justice. One difference is that rather than planetary level, the base of the pyramid is governmental responsibility and policies. The top of the pyramid is individual in terms of understanding, delivering, looking after one's health. In that context the funding of the NHS and where it should lie becomes an interesting question.

NC: Well, the first thing you need to do is decide what you wanted to do. I mean, don't turn it into a financial question. It is astonishing how quickly people turn a health issue into a financial question. They decide how they're going to fund it, but haven't decided what it's going to do.

I: One of the big tragedies of Western medicine has been this mind-body dualism. That can create problems for communities and patients and increases stigma and discrimination and all that. How do we bring physical and mental health together?

NC: It is not just about public health. I don't think we should segment it. It's everyone's responsibility, not only public health doctors responsible? Actually, it's about businesses, it's about schools, it's about all the institutions that shape our lives. And if the government were to focus on how can they motivate and mobilise those people? And it's about creating health. It's not simply about prevention, but about creating health. If people are resilient, confident and competent, they will be better able to shrug off infections. We know that they will also be better able to make sensible decisions about food and alcohol and sex and driving their car too fast and everything else that adds chaos as well as excitement to life. So I really would start in a different place. I think the big two levers for change are political will to mobilise the community and changing professional education. In the meantime the NHS will just carry on. I would not shift its funding. I would encourage its leaders to make improvements like surgical hubs which are good but not strategic. Those changes are about survival. So the change will come over the next 10–15 years but only if politicians are willing to grasp this wider notion of health. That's about all of us. And at the same time if the educators are willing to grasp the idea that actually professional education has gone in a poor direction and that they need to be thinking much harder about exactly the mind-body Cartesian split and how it has worked or not worked and the link between the individual, the community, the society and the planet. Therefore, your successors as doctors are going to have something different inside their heads, which is not simply about the bones of the foot or being a saviour but focused on their skills which can help facilitate other people.

I: There are major challenges in education as we keep adding to the curriculum without taking anything away. You have already touched upon professional education, can you expand on that?

NC: Yes. There is a report that was produced in 2010 about the future of health professional education for the 21st century which was written by a group chaired by Julio Frank and Lincoln Chen. Julio Frank was minister of health in Mexico and dean of public health at Harvard, and he's now president of Miami University. And Lincoln Chen was president of the Chinese Medical Foundation. And they had a group of people including Richard Horton and me. I was the only non-clinician on the entire thing, but it came up with some really sensible stuff which has to be competence based and to start weaving an understanding of the system with an understanding of the body. But it also came up with something which I thought was really helpful. This was the three stages of education. There is the informative– when you learn about the body systems, the basics, and that enables you to become a specialist. Then there are the formative bits where that is added to behaviours and values and one becomes a professional. Then there is the transformative bit, and that's when one can become a leader and also an agent of change, as they described it at the time. For Julio as a public health doctor, it was a fascinating exercise during Covid, to manage a whole population of students and faculty at Miami University. He observed that when it comes to professional education, the learning of body systems can be done as well if and perhaps better through technology and it need not be in person. So two years or whatever to learn all the foundation and maybe two years at university to do the formative bit to put it into more real life situations – learning how to make decisions with this knowledge, relating to patients and society and so on – followed by transformative learning in the workplace. This is a very different approach to the current process of professional education because the content, particularly in the second bit, would cover a lot of the social and economic determinants and so on. You can do some of that over the Internet, but some of that needs to be face to face where you're confronting differences and seeing things differently. In some ways you can't deal with prejudice unless you have something more authentic than just reading books about it or doing lectures on it. Our report to be published tomorrow is called Probable Futures and Radical Possibilities. And the Probable Futures are the bits where we have talked to people all over the world and there is a sort of consensus that the future will have blended services dipping in and out for caring for the children in person. Depending on the circumstances, it's going to be a future where people have closer links between specialties and a future more focused on primary care. Then our radical possibilities include, for example, changing professional education, thereby creating a different kind of professional, but doing things in different ways, which may well be cheaper, but also more accessible. One of our other radical possibilities is we looked at in Cuba, the Latin American medical school, which deliberately only takes in people from poor communities. So you and I cannot apply. It takes deliberately indigenous people who then go back and work within their own communities. Another thing that we are again advocating is that we should be making the paths into professionalism much more open to more people. And that doesn't mean getting more people into Oxford and Cambridge yet, which of course is fine. In the end, not everyone goes to Oxford and Cambridge or indeed to the rest of universities but making pathways that are different. So these are some of our radical possibilities. So you'll gather that in a way I am not terribly interested in talking about the NHS. I am commenting from outside and with a wider societal focus.

I: What you are proposing is a new vision and if the NHS were not to look at it, it would be in deeper trouble than it is. We know that gaps in the workforce exist which affect people's wellbeing. We do need to do things differently. We cannot carry on the same way. That brings me back to your vision as a disruptor. We do need disruptors from time to time to sort of shake things up and the kaleidoscope can readjust, but there are multiple factors. How do we integrate care? Increased specialisation is good in lots of ways but it does make care for the patients very very difficult. And that goes back to one of your original reports about generalism versus specialism.

NC: Yes, where we confront that in our report is very much about giving people a broader base in education. We were following the GMC report about five years ago so that there is a broader base so that you understand more of it and also competency based. There is also something I remember when I was working in Oxford 25 years ago, there was quite a lot of debate about people trying to hang on to general physicians. Every cardiologist was going to be an interventional cardiologist rather than a physician cardiologist. And some of the research at that point pointed out that it was about teams being organised in certain ways but also having other specialists. The best care was provided by a general physician team which had specialists as part of the firm. The question is not whether you are cared for by general physicians or specialists. There are two issues here... the first is educational but there is also the organisational bit. That is about teams – their constituents and functions of individuals. Also, how often GPs get involved in hospital teams? That should be the norm.

I: I suppose something like telehealth could change that.

NC: That's absolutely right. I'm sure it could.

I: Using technology, GPs could join the ward round when their patient was being discussed.

NC: Yes, that would be great. I think that's a very good example of how technology could really enable this stuff in real time. If they were not able to do so, they could be given a very short video.

I: There are interesting examples from the US where from rural areas, patients record their symptoms and send them on to psychiatric teams who study it and then work with the patients to help manage their symptoms. There appears to be a degree of reluctance, particularly in medical profession, about sharing education across disciplines.

NC: There is no reason why that that first two years of specialist knowledge shouldn't be for any one even laypeople doing it through these Massive Open Online Course (MOOC) methods online. So these modules from centres of excellence will help share specialist knowledge and people can go as far as they can go simply because some people will not be able to grasp some of the more complex concepts of biochemistry but they could grasp other aspects such as statistics, which you also need. So that doesn't mean to say people shouldn't all just start off with understanding how a particular body system works. You know, how you know why a muscle contracts. Some of that is very basic and terribly simple, whereas other bits can be complex just for professionals. I think there's massive scope for that.

I: I think in a roundabout way, we've covered everything.

NC: I'm afraid I've been a bit troublesome.

I: I think you're absolutely spot on. I feel that we keep reinventing the wheel. We have to do things differently. Society has changed, people's expectations have changed and if we are not changing services in line with what's available then we are in serious trouble. The point that you make about technology is an incredibly important one.

NC: I think there are huge opportunities with the technology. But if one recognises that health is determined about 70% outside the health system, whatever the exact number is, then actually we should focus on that. Only 20–30% is inside the health system and all the conversation is about that but fiddling with that proportion is not going to change the 70–80%. If we get an epidemic of diabetes or depression or addictions then the NHS may be able to pick up the pieces well or badly, but it isn't going to affect the causes. So who's going to affect the causes? I think it's much more about networks and nodes and so on. As an individual I have a whole series of people I'm close to in different sorts of ways. I'm close to institutions in many different sorts of ways. And we are terribly lucky in that we can reach out to people in completely different ways. We take it on a human level of these sorts of social, economic and other networks. And I have a slightly old fashioned view. This is about humanity. This is about values. This is about not getting too over-done on the specialisms because, of course, you want them when you want them but most of health is not about that.

I: Is there anything else that you would like to add that we have not covered? It's been absolutely fabulous.

NC: I think I've given you my views. Yes. I mean, it's been really fasci-nating for a number of reasons because I think there is a lot to be done. There are major challenges for the NHS and I'm not sure that anybody is actually looking at it. It is very much a kind of Band Aid and lurching from crisis to crisis rather than saying that we need to sit down and discuss with the punters and the stakeholders and ask what kind of health service you want and how do we develop and deliver that? Going back to the ideas of creation of health rather than treating illnesses is the correct way forward.

NC: I suspect but I don't know. In the Indian tradition, there will be some interesting things that we could learn from around this and certainly in Chinese tradition as well, I would have thought.

I: The Ayurvedic tradition does not believe in mind-body dualism. Mind and body influence each other and are affected by factors like diet and environment and weather which affect your health. Often people will use multiple healthcare systems.

NC: And the trouble with something like the NHS is you start off with an existing body with existing ways of doing things. If I were a health minister I would encourage them to get on with it and to keep making improvements and keep the pressure on. I would con-centrate my efforts for improvement outside the NHS, including in professional education. I suspect there's money to be saved on professional education too actually.

I: We really need to look at how we educate. As I said, we are still educating medical students as if it's the 1950s. I think that that is a real tragedy. Thank you so much for your time. You have given some truly wonderful ideas. Really appreciate it.

4 Sir Ian Gilmore

Sir Ian Gilmore is a Professor of hepatology, director of the Liverpool Centre for Alcohol Research, and chair of the Alcohol Health Alliance. He is currently an advisor to the Royal College of Physicians of London on alcohol. He is also the past president of the Royal College of Physicians. He trained at Cambridge University and St Thomas' Hospital, qualifying in 1971 and subsequently specialising in gastroenterology, specifically liver disease. He was Chair of Liverpool Health Partners from 2013– to 2017 and currently chairs Liverpool Foundation NHS Trust. He has published widely on alcohol and liver diseases.

Interview

I: What is your view of the NHS at the present time?

IG: As has been stated many times in newspaper headlines, the NHS is in crisis, but it has been for the last 50+ years. So, what is the current crisis? Is it a bigger crisis or just a different perspective – seeing it now away from the frontline and when a lot of one's experiences are second-hand coming from friends and relatives who may not be medical but are using the NHS. But, to be honest, it does seem to be on a downward trajectory and it is not a result of Covid that the service is not coping. For example, I know that there are services that should have 12 acute physicians but are running with only 6, putting a tremendous amount of strain on those doctors. So, it is not a good place to be. I worry. I do worry about people in acute medicine and in A&E. And of course my own advancing years bring increasing personal anxiety about the preparedness of the NHS, I have to say.

I: Looking back, do you think was there ever a golden age?

IG: Looking back, I feel there was but also doubt whether it was really fair. My experience has been entirely in hospital medicine, and there was almost certainly a lot of racial and gender discrimination. The consultants often promoted individuals on criteria that

DOI: 10.4324/9781003382188-4

wouldn't pass transparency tests. But on the other hand, the system seemed to work in the sense that juniors worked incredibly hard, and they felt that they were working towards a nirvana. They were working towards a time when they would not be so much in the front line but be more in a supervisory role. And that's gone now. It's very hard to put it into words because there were things that were not right then. One wants to avoid being an old fuddy-duddy with rose-tinted spectacles, particularly one that is male, pale and stale! But there's no doubt at all that the breakdown of the firm structure within hospitals has destroyed the corporate spirit. Junior doctors, even when ill, did not take time off as they knew that it was their colleagues who would have to pick up the load. Now sickness rates have risen because often juniors are unaware who it is that they're letting down. They see that as the problem of the HR (Human Resources) who have to dig up a locum who doesn't know the hospital but wanders in and gets paid a lot. So, I think the hospital system has changed since doctors' hours were limited by the EU Directive. Now, I'm not saying that we should go back to 120 hours a week, but I know it has been quite hard to train in some surgical specialties, for example, when the trainees are not able to put in the hours. I think some juniors would prefer to work more hours in exchange for more genuine training opportunities to build up their skills. I am not putting this forward as a solution to the workforce crisis, but I wonder, now that we are no longer in the European Union, if there is some scope to look at getting a better balance between time at work and genuine training.

I: Do you think that the old apprenticeship model worked better in terms of training?

IG: I suspect it still is an apprentice model in many ways, but the model does not work so well because of the fragmentation of the way hospital services are provided. I think the apprenticeship model has got a long and venerable history. There is something about working with an experienced colleague that aids the understanding and development of the ability to manage risk and handle the unknown. In a system under strain, this is more essential than ever and probably distinguishes doctors from other healthcare workers. It is very difficult to put into words where that's learnt. But I think the apprenticeship system, working alongside more experienced colleagues, is part of that.

I: Do you think the NHS is fit for purpose as it stands?

IG: No, I don't think it is. I think it's failing a lot of people at the moment. There are still inequalities of access that shouldn't be there. I think that clearly it is not fit for its purpose when waiting lists, for example for cancer treatments, are the way they are and when people are waiting several years for joint replacement, etc. No, it isn't. It isn't fit for purpose at present.

I: So, what do you think needs to change?

IG: Well, I think there are obviously short-term and long-term aspects that have to change. Workforce is the main urgency, partly because it takes so long for proper remedies to the workforce. And I think that's what Andrew Goddard (President of the Royal College of Physicians of London at the time of the interview) has been very articulate and persistent in emphasizing. In the short term, we undoubtedly need more support workers, such as physician associates and specialist nurses. I have found that they work best in quite narrow fields where they can get up to speed relatively quickly. I would rather have a specialist nurse in hepatology in the clinic alongside me than an SpR (Specialist Registrar) who has just rotated from cardiology. I feel it is more challenging to put physician associates or specialist nurses in A&E department or a general clinic with unselected patients. I think it can work, provided doctors embrace taking on people in new roles to work with them, and I don't think that all doctors are doing that yet. Sometimes, staff get thrown in at the deep end without induction. Support staff with training and mentoring can be a really good asset as they slowly become more independent. I think we as a profession could do better in preparing them for filling support roles. We know that the pharmacists can give excellent advice but inevitably look through the lens of medication without broader training. And so, yes, certainly in the short term, we need to expand the role of others to work with doctors. But I think doctors have to be prepared to take on more responsibility in supervising them. That takes time away from what they would be doing otherwise. But if we don't do it, I think we all are going to suffer the consequences. So, that is the workforce side. But obviously, there are a lot of other challenges in providing a healthcare system, particularly when funding is tight. I am personally of the view that fragmentation of the system is one of the biggest problems. But how does one square the circle of having a joined-up national system but with some devolved responsibility to local areas? Because if everything is dictated centrally, people locally lose interest and don't feel valued. On the other hand, I think if local services such as, in my own area of interest, addiction services, are contracted out to the lowest bidder, it can be catastrophic. I do want to see the NHS take control for health and social care, but it needs to be done in a nuanced way that there is local support. It is amazing the way that local populations come together in times of crises. Undoubtedly, there's a wealth of support in local communities for the older people and so on, if one could get it packaged right. I don't know how we do it, but I think that it is a priority. We are not going to succeed unless we do manage to get local buy-in to the system. And I don't think people feel any great buy-in to their local healthcare at the moment. Their perception is of an A+E 8-hour wait to be seen, then perhaps a 24-hour trolley wait and GPs that seem increasingly difficult to see. I am no expert on the history and workings of the GP as an independent contractor, but I understand there is a debate within General Practice as to whether GPs should sit more firmly within the NHS. Many younger GPs seem happy to be salaried rather than independent contractors. Social care clearly is another huge part of the jigsaw that has been disrupted recently. I know you want to talk about patients and the contract between doctors and society as well. I don't think we can just solve social care with more money, although undoubtedly it would help. We do need to somehow rebalance that contract and people's feelings towards the local healthcare system.

I: You touched upon a lot of things that I was going to pick up later on anyway. If you were in a position and had the power to redesign the NHS, what would the model look like?

IG: Well, I think, the model should be joined up and with clearer pathways of care. This needs health and social care to be joined up, whether through community care coming under an acute trust or whether you have some other model. I would also bring public health back into the NHS, although it is a difficult one. I think there have been some benefits in having directors of public health sitting in city councils. I would perhaps develop a more hybrid model, but I think we've lost something with public health sitting outside the NHS. I have always been a proponent of public health doctors retaining some clinical work and that model does work in some places. I think for a public health doctor to do a clinic once a week helps keep their feet on the ground, just as I think it's crazy that when there are 12 cardiologists appointing a 13th cardiologist, to appoint another interventional cardiologist instead of someone to take an interest in the epidemiology of cardiovascular disease in their catchment and extrapolate it to community education and prevention. I think we need to integrate public health better. Of course, we need to integrate psychiatry better, and it sometimes feels that psychiatry has wandered off into another planet from the rest of medicine. I would like to try to re-integrate psychiatry a bit more. I think the trust system has caused increased fragmentation in the NHS. Recently, I was at a hospital that had four separate trusts within that one hospital. There was a cardiothoracic trust, a mental health trust, a general hospital trust and one other I've forgotten. They all just built their drawbridges and dug their moats. There has been some moving back on that by fusing trusts, but it has not been always welcome because some of the smaller specialist trusts have benefited from the independence but at the expense of the general trusts. And that's been a particular problem where I work in Liverpool, which is unique in the number of specialist trusts such as obstetrics and gynaecology, children's health, cardiothoracic, neurology, cancer and psychiatry. But it has not worked for the central teaching hospital that was left bereft of crucial specialist services on site. My vision would be to have a national health service, but with genuine local control and more opportunities for local communities to contribute in ways like local health champions and supporting the elderly in their own homes. But I don't have an answer for how to do it. We are going to get onto the social contract. But, you know, we are where we are, where people feel that if they are unwell, something needs to be done about it and quickly. When did you start working in the NHS?

I: In 1979 or thereabouts.

IG: I was only half a dozen or so years ahead of you. For the first ten years or so as a consultant, the families of patients rarely asked to see me about their loved one in the hospital, whereas now they are queuing up to see the consultant, often less than happy with the care being given. In those early days, patients still remembered the pre-NHS era and felt almost inappropriately grateful for the care they got. Inappropriately in my view because the people remembered what it was like before the NHS and so they felt they were getting something for nothing, even though they were paying through general taxation. They felt privileged to get treatment rather than as their right. Changing attitudes are inevitable 75 years into the NHS, expectations are understandably different and have not been helped by successive recent governments not doing well in engendering trust or funding the rapidly expanding therapeutic possibilities.

I: There is the issue of patients' rights versus responsibilities and how do we manage that? Smoking and alcohol spring to mind.

IG: I think those are good examples. I don't blame the alcohol-dependent patient or the patient who is hooked on nicotine. I blame the system that allowed them to get there as the power of global industry has steamrollered governments. The problem is prevention requires fundamental attitudinal change. We would be a happier and better society with much more prevention. But I'm not sure that it'd be any cheaper, because, whatever happens, you consume most of your healthcare costs in the last few years of life, and death is inevitable.

I: One of the other things that has shifted in the last 25–30 years is a generational shift in attitudes to work–life balance. Therefore, workforce planning in that sense also creates additional problems. We are also getting a generation of people who are coming to the clinic with printouts from the net and saying that they want drug A, B or C. And there has been a very limited dialogue on that. How do you think we can shift that and have a more open discussion not only with the patients and their carers but also with the younger generation of workforce.

IG: Well, we haven't touched on social and health inequalities much yet, but there's no doubt that narrower the gap in social inequalities, the healthier and happier the population is. I always look back fondly at Scandinavian countries because I was brought up in Newcastle upon Tyne and as a schoolboy could take a boat for £8 return to Esbjerg Denmark and hitchhike around Denmark, Sweden and Norway. I think these countries still have some of the narrowest gaps in inequalities and are still amongst the heathiest and happiest countries. They operate a form of National Health Service reasonably successfully. I'm sure there are pressures in those countries too, but until we in the UK can narrow that gap in social and health inequalities through better access to education and a fairer society, I think we're going to struggle in the balance between individual responsibility for health and the role of the state in providing healthcare.

I: You have touched upon the idea of social contract. How do you think we can try and build on that? People keep demanding more and more investigations and more and more expensive interventions, and yet there seems to be a reluctance to pay for it. So, somebody's got to pay for it. How do we convince them?

IG: A very good question. I get a bit depressed that the only discussion one really sees in the media about death is assisted dying and physician-assisted suicide. Everybody is going to die. And I think we need to somehow open up that discussion. We know that most people would like to die at home yet most die in hospital. Patients and their families understand the generalities of life and death from a philosophical view but as soon as we are ill, we want a solution. It usually needs a hospital and often expensive chemotherapy, even though it may prolong life by only a few weeks and often make you feel pretty ill at the same time. I don't have solutions and probably will be the same when it is my turn. There is no doubt that expectations are raised by the media, who will pick one or two cases that make the point they want to make. I do think we need to try to engage the public more in their health, and I think we have to do that when they're well, because it's very difficult to engage people when they are ill: when they are seeking solutions at any cost and with a pre-set mind. Having a society that is more health-literate is more likely to be able to engage in a proper debate, and this brings us back to narrowing the inequality gap.

I: Again, in the context of Scandinavia, there are obviously lessons from there. I am not sure why are we reluctant to learn from them? Is it simply the numbers are massive here and Scandinavian countries have smaller populations or is it something else?

IG: It may be an accident of history as much as anything else. We were a leading industrial country that needed workers, coal miners and others. We also had colonies and an empire that gave us delusions of grandeur. We probably were a more polarised society than the Scandinavian ones for hundreds of years, with our landowners and professions distinct from the workers. So, it takes a long time to reverse those sorts of things. But it is a fact that the Scandinavians do have the narrowest gap, I suspect because they started off with better cards than the UK did.

I: You touched upon the question of training and in particular across disciplines and the role of a physician assistant and nurse specialists. Is there a model you think that we can bring the groups together, including medical students and trainees to try and start off with a common learning basis and then people wander off into their specialties? Is there any mileage in that?

IG: I think the more people share their training and their experiences in study and outside study, the better a system will work. Undoubtedly, there is still an arrogance amongst doctors that doctors know best. On the other hand, there may have been a decline in the status of nursing. When I was a student at St Thomas's hospital, for many nurses in training, it was a kind of finishing school for ladies – but I suspect that was the case particularly in the teaching hospitals of the day. There have been changes in the demographics of other branches of healthcare professionals too. I don't know how greater integration of training would work in our healthcare system, but I am sure there will be models elsewhere worth examining. I do think that joint learning breaks down barriers and any 'us and them' mentality, but I don't see it as a fundamental problem in the NHS that people don't work together. I think by and large when you throw people together as in operating theatres or in primary care, they do work together, and the current problem is the tsunami of work and the pressures that brings. As I said earlier, there is a challenge in getting doctors to embrace the roles that other healthcare professionals can take. Working with them and helping them to take on more advanced roles and to take on some of the work, the doctors often do this but they have to be given the time. We can't just devolve medical work to others but throw them unsupported into the deep end.

I: As Covid has illustrated, there is a major degree of goodwill and altruism in the community. One of the things that really fascinated me was that right at the beginning of the pandemic when the prime minister asked for 250,000 volunteers and 750,000 did volunteer.

So, what happened to those 500,000? Why do you think we are not using that social capital to go back to and support the communities?

IG: Indeed

I: Also, as you were saying, it is about setting national standards but local delivery – how do we bring that shift in? Can we facilitate change in that?

IG: Well, it is perhaps the only good thing Andrew Lansley did in his reforms was to try to take health out of politics, but he failed. It was always destined to fail and actually ended up making the system worse by separating NHS England from the Department of Health. Health is so important to individuals that I think it's always going to be a political football and needs a minister to stand up in Parliament to defend it. And I think we have to accept that. But we still shouldn't stop looking for ways to kind of protect local services from central control. Of course, Foundation Trusts tried to do that but when you speak to the CEOs of Foundation Trusts, they are under more direct pressure, for example with phone calls from the Secretary of State on a Friday afternoon saying why is your waiting list so long. Although I have no solutions jumping up at me, I do think that we need to look at ways that the NHS can be more successfully devolved to local management. Perhaps the Integrated Care Systems and Boards being set up may help but we must ensure they are not just Regional Health Authorities under another name.

I: The pandemic has shown that we can do lots of telehealth so how do we sort this out in training and delivery of services and utilise technologies? And what would your advice be in terms of getting it right?

IG: Well, if you put the patient at the centre, you have the chance to get it right. I have been very impressed by the system in my own general practice. This form of telephone triage has been used for the last four or five years and it works very well. I think the success there is that because doctors who are phoning up the patient are experienced and often know the patient. They are not trying to keep patients away, rather seeing what's the best solution for that individual person. And so, they're not prescribing antibiotics over the phone, but saying if somebody might have an infection, come in and we will see you today.

Telemedicine is fine and a lot of routine follow-up can be done that way. But again, it needs even more experience than face-to-face contact, in particular picking up when a physical examination may be needed. I suppose that doctors of my era who spent hours peering at the jugular venous pressure or trying to decide if there was fixed splitting of the second heart sound lament the passing of the primacy of the physical examination. But when an echocardiogram can answer the same questions and more, perhaps we just have to move on, provided we can train our successors to judge when to order an echo from subtle hints at the teleconsultation. There is little doubt that over-investigation, already an issue driven by fear of litigation, is likely to be made worse by the added uncertainty of a telephone or video-consultation. Perhaps we're not educating people to work in that way well enough and need more research, more evidence and better implementation of telemedicine.

I: One of the things that strikes me is how bad the NHS is at work-force planning. With around 60% of medical students being female and as mentioned earlier with the generational shift of attitudes towards work–life balance, there seems to be no understanding of these shifting demographics. Both the staff and patient demographics are changing. What do you think we ought to be doing now?

IG: As I said earlier, junior doctors were prepared to sweat through a very tough system because they could see nirvana on the horizon when they became a consultant or a partner in a general practice, that life would be tolerable and they would have time for their family, get their holidays and so on. I think the problem now is that the juniors are still under the cosh, but they can't see light at the end of the tunnel, if I can freely mix my metaphors. If you look at law and you've got any friends whose children are starting off in the solicitors' offices, you will know they're often working 18 hours a day. No European Working Time Directive for them but they do long hours because when they reach partner status, they know that there will be another generation of youngsters doing the hard groundwork. Our experiences 30 years ago in medicine could not be justified on safety grounds, where the juniors learnt the hard way when consultants were a rare sight at evenings and weekends. But there is a balance to be struck and I think we need to get better at modifying consultant roles as they get older. In my career, I have witnessed several surgeons who clearly lost their appetite and probably their nerve for operating when they reached their late 50s and early 60s. In general, we've been very bad at adapting doctors' working patterns as they get older. And that is perhaps why they walk out at 60. So, I think there's a lot that could be done over retention in the NHS. And if we don't do it, I think there will be a bigger crisis before long – if that is possible. So, I think that's really important. How would one do that in a very complex system? It would require the government to accept that it was crucial and undertake to implement the outcome of an independent review. The task of the review would be to really look at the ways that current roles could be made more fulfilling not only for those who are just qualifying and are full of ideals and ambitions and want to look after patients but also for retention of senior staff. It certainly isn't just about money.

I: In a series of studies, we found that the rates of burnout among medical students and doctors are truly massive. I do not know what we are doing to these very bright, young, energetic, enthusiastic medical students. One of the interesting things that some medical students said to me in person was that they don't like the idea of simulation, and they had not come into medicine to be technicians. Simulation made them feel that at the back of their mind they know that the person in front of them is an actor and they're being paid for it. So, how do they generate that empathy? How do we resolve that?

IG: I don't know much about medical student selection now, and I am sure it has moved on from the parochial days when the two questions that were asked to get into a London teaching hospital were: Where did your father train and what position do you play? But your feedback on current student attitudes to simulation are interesting and needs to be heeded. There has to be a balance and it would be unacceptable to allow students to put in intravenous cannulae without practicing on a dummy arm first. Also, role play in areas like medical ethics can be a lot more interesting and educational than a dry lecture.

I: I think it reflects the need for other talents which helps one to become a team player and learn from each other and an ability to relax, having a sense of humour to cope. What is your view on integration of health and social care and mental and physical health?

IG: Yes, absolutely. I do think that somehow joining up health and social care is important. And I also think that giving more opportunities for local involvement is crucial. Volunteering makes people feel a pride in the local healthcare. On the background of Michael Marmot's work on social determinants, we must do something about the widening gap.

I: I think you're absolutely right. There is often no integration between different branches of medicine in acute care and mental health and social care and public health. But it's also linking health with other things like education, employment, housing and justice. We just can't see health in isolation. That is maybe one of the tragedies. I don't know anywhere in the world where there is a kind of interconnected way. Often, the Department of Health does not talk to anyone.

IG: That's right. The Department of Health and Social Care lurches from crisis to crisis, mirroring what is going on in the field. One feeds off the other, and there seems no prospect of breaking that cycle any time soon. Sorry to end on a pessimistic note!

I: Absolutely. That is all from my side. Really appreciate it.

IG: Thanks very much.

5   Dr Sarah Hallett

Dr Sarah Hallett is a paediatrician in training. She has been joint chair of Junior Doctors Committee of the BMA. In this role, she has led on advocating for junior doctors. She is actively involved in improving working conditions for junior doctors.

Interview

I: Thanks very much for making the time. NHS of the future is going to affect your generation more in lots of ways so the focus really is about the next few decades of the health service. Shall we kick off with your views on the strengths and weaknesses of the NHS as it stands. If you had the power, what would you do differently? What is your vision?

SH: It is a huge question. I think the strengths of the NHS from the start has been a model and as a philosophy to ensure that members of our society are able to access world-class healthcare that is free at the point of access to overall keep our population healthy, which then in turn makes economic sense. And those principles, I think, still stand and should still be respected. When you compare it with other countries, the fact is that a disparate point of views and accessibility is a huge strength of the NHS. And I think that is what makes many of us proud to work for it. Tragically obviously we focus a lot on the problems that the NHS is facing and that is the very nature of how we operate. We are always going to find problems and try to fix these. I have talked a lot in various different fora about how underfunded the NHS is, how overstretched it is and the challenges that we face in the NHS on a daily basis. I also feel that we don't celebrate enough the positives that the NHS has and the work its staff put in rather concentrate on its negatives. We do not celebrate the staff enough perhaps because there is a tendency to believe that private is good and public bad. People who work in the NHS are inherently people who have chosen to do so because they do

DOI: 10.4324/9781003382188-5

want to help other people. So they are one of its greatest resources. But the issues and the problems that they face are often not well-managed at all. NHS is about care from preconception all the way through to almost after death. And the NHS caters for incredibly rare conditions, for example, recent advances in spinal muscular atrophy treatments for young babies. We are able as a nation to manage these because of the fact we have a national healthcare service, we are able to lobby and get the world-class treatments that people in other countries are having to pay millions of pounds (or equivalent) for. I think that's an incredible strength of the service. It is just a fantastic organisation in general. Of course, it has weaknesses too and often these are out of the control of those who work in it. It has been underfunded chronically and overstretched. And we are currently experiencing the greatest staffing and workforce crisis that the NHS has ever faced. The Health and Social Care Select Committee produced a report on this recently which stated in no uncertain terms that we are facing the greatest workforce crisis the NHS has ever faced and the resource being put into the NHS is nowhere near enough to deal with that. We also have known for a considerable period of time that there have been no meaningful attempts at workforce planning. A decade or so ago, the Centre for Workforce Intelligence was predicting the number of consultants we needed, notwithstanding that most of their predictions were wrong, nevertheless, there doesn't appear to have been any meaningful attempts to rectify that since the Centre for Workforce Intelligence stopped existing. We are training more medical students than we have been before, but it's not near as many as organisations like the Royal College of Physicians are projecting that we need. They did produce a report which called for a doubling in the number of medical students. And so we are far off that. Paradoxically and interestingly there is no commitment to jobs as junior doctors for those medical students once they graduate. We can train as many medical students as we want but unless we are willing to put them in jobs, then it is entirely pointless. Medical unemployment would be a disaster when we have a real need for more doctors. The other issue that we have is that we do not have the actual statistics for those doctors who leave, where they leave from, where they go to, at what level, what specialty, why did they leave, do they migrate or leave medicine altogether, etc. There has been academic work done looking at training numbers but we do not know what happens to doctors once they get into the training system. We do have data about recruitment, but we don't have any data about retention. So we are not able to make any meaningful progress unless and until we have that data. We cannot really plan services if we do not know how many people are going to come in and stay and continue to provide services in the short, medium and long terms. One of the other potential weaknesses that we have in the NHS is that very often we are firefighting. We are fighting against impacts that have been inflicted on patients in other parts of their lives. There is that fantastic quote about the fact that medicine is politics on a larger scale by Virchow. I feel very strongly and often I do think when I'm seeing patients in A&E or elsewhere, that actually I could make a bigger difference to their lives as a politician than I can as a doctor. As a paediatrician, the impact on the children that I see are as a result of wider societal and public health factors choices made by the government which result in poverty, poor housing, underfunding Sure Start centres, reducing support for mothers, limited or poor peri-natal care when social services are incredibly stretched so I have concerns about children, who are the future generations and the impact on their health and consequently on the society. As a clinician I know that community support can be very difficult to get. Similar issues emerge at the other end of life with the elderly who need care packages and the support in the community. What we see as happening with the energy crisis will hugely impact upon pensioners where pensions are not keeping pace with inflation and cost of living is going up. As doctors, we see the fallout of that at work every day. As the NHS is reliant on funding from politicians, we have every reason to and ought to expect them to make sensible decisions about all areas of policy, whether it is education, housing, employment, energy and even design of cities. These are all interconnected. I do think that the NHS has been underfunded and is overstretched, but I also think wider policy decisions that have been made by the government in recent years have also acted to undermine what the NHS is able to do for patients and the public. Furthermore, all of this has been further compounded by the various different Acts or so-called reforms being pushed through the parliament to change the way that we organise the NHS. I believe very strongly that the private sector should not be involved in the NHS because I believe it wastes money. It undermines the NHS because private providers tend to cherry pick the patients that they take from the NHS that tend to make it more expensive for the rest of the NHS to operate. And if things go wrong in the private sector patients then get shunted back to the NHS for acute care. The marketisation of the NHS ultimately will undermine the structure of how we deliver care as well.

I: Thanks, that is very helpful and clear about the challenges faced by the NHS. If you were the health minister and you had the power to redesign the NHS, what would you do differently?

SH: One of my first plans would be workforce planning because we are unable to do anything without a sensible people plan. And I know there have been attempts made at developing people plans, but they have not gone far enough in terms of workforce planning. I would want to ensure we had a proper workforce strategy that was fully funded. I would go to the Treasury and I would be asking the Chancellor for more money for the NHS. I think it makes economic sense. No matter which part of the political spectrum he sits on, having a healthy working population is only good for our economy. The money that is invested in the NHS therefore works its way back into the wider economy. We need to be increasing the number of training posts that we have for doctors. As a profession and as a society, we need to have a conversation about other healthcare professionals and their roles and responsibilities too. I personally feel that once we have filled all of the gaps that exist in the medical workforce, we may end up with further bottlenecks that prevent progression. I do think there is a role for medical associate professionals in the NHS and I think we need to have a conversation about that and which is not protectionist of the doctors as a profession. We are not going to be replaced as a profession, but there are benefits to working more closely with other healthcare professionals helping us. I do think that physician associates are highly qualified individuals who probably would want job progression as well. Some of their work will be clinical at ward level, others may well be in the community so we need a sensible discussion about that. There are other special issues. For example, women's health strategy has been published recently. But it must come to fruition. I do have a declaration of interest that obviously being a woman but I also feel that we are potentially letting down a large subsection of our society. I realise that is just the way that politics works. The way the politicians and politics see the NHS is not necessarily the most efficient way. The fact that we have had three health secretaries in the past few months says something. This also reflects importance or lack thereof given to health. The politicians come and they go and do not necessarily make any decisions for which they may be held accountable in the long term. Of course, they obviously have very good civil servants who are able to advise them. But politicians need to learn how to listen as well. They (politicians) need some experience of the health service. The fact that it can just be people brought in with no experience in the health service just because it is politically convenient for that particular Prime Minister to have them in the Cabinet, is really staggering and disappointing. No NHS staff would be appointed that way. This is one of the most important roles that exists in the NHS because of the political and organisational structures. I would look to find ways to mitigate that. The Secretary of State has major power over the work of the NHS, whether they have had any experience of health service or not. I wouldn't be in favour of removing the NHS out of political control because I think the NHS is a political organisation. Huge amounts of funding as a nation goes towards it which also makes it a political football. While it can be used as a political football, I don't think it should be taken outside of politics, but I do think that the political control should be pragmatic and needs to be levelled out with people who actually do have experience in that area. Another reason for keeping that control is health's link with education, housing, employment, etc. which lie with other ministries so a seat on the table helps the NHS.

I: What are your views about integration of physical and mental health, health and social care?

SH: I think examples like the Bromley-by-Bow Centre for integration of social health with the physical health is a really good model and one that could be followed by services across the rest of the NHS. (This is done through social prescribing.) As I said earlier, we are constantly firefighting in the NHS. There needs to be proper funding for these schemes across different fields through local authorities or central government, and the NHS has a role in being involved in that. As Sure Start centres and groups supporting people with their daily lives and keeping people healthy have shown it is important to deliver these in an interconnected manner. The NHS has a role to play in preventive medicine in that way and kind of social medicine as it were. Health has to be connected with public health in an integrated manner.

I: As we talked about it earlier, it is a real tragedy that health is seen in a silo but it isn't. You were saying quite rightly, that, you are seeing children and you patch them up and send them back to sometimes hideous places to live in and not surprisingly they fail to thrive.

SH: Yeah.

I: One of the things that really intrigues me as a clinician is the tension between patients' rights and responsibilities, and how do we deal with these?

SH: It is partly about education. There does come a point when some of these narratives can almost put too much on patients in terms of saying, things like you should eat healthily or do more exercise well, which may be fine in theory. But these messages and pressures often ignore the reality of the situations that many members of our society are actually living in. So we may be putting more demands on people who are living in poverty and these messages make them feel bullied. Cooking a fresh, healthy meal from scratch is a lot more challenging if somebody does not have a well-stocked kitchen, a well-stocked fridge and perhaps the ability to afford ingredients or even pay for gas or electricity. There are so many other things that someone may need to just keep their head above water. I do believe that the NHS can educate patients around what they can expect (from the service). I think there is also some expectation in management that needs to be done but in a way that also acknowledges the privileges that some of us have that many of our patients often don't. That means more and better working with patients from those kinds of demographic groups is incredibly important because sometimes it is difficult for us to imagine the challenges they face in their daily lives. Also, worth remembering that even patients who are involved in our management structures are often a self-selecting group who engage with us on those levels. So it is about making sure we're reaching those unheard voices of our patients out there to ensure that our services are what they need. In turn, that will allow us to understand what their challenges are so that when we provide that (specific) education, we can realistically manage their expectations of the NHS but it is also about managing society's expectations. Again, a lot of this is political choice. For example, GPs are currently getting a lot of blame for appointment times and how difficult it is to see a GP and facing the ire of the patients. The reality is that GPs can only work with the funding and the resources that they have been given by the government. So some education on the facts will be helpful. Politicians have a very limited vision as they care about votes and getting re-elected which is another problem. It means that the government thinks very short term as they think about the next five years. They don't think about what is happening in 50 years' time. Realistically they don't even think about the next five years, because at 18-month point they start getting ready for the next general election and next term. So really when it comes to the NHS, we need to be thinking 30, or 40 or even 50 years down the line, not about the next couple of years. I think patient engagement is the key through patient education but it has to be done in a very sensible and sensitive way. We know from Michael Marmot's health gap work that health is a gradient. It is not about poverty and riches but people in the middle who are living in different gradients. These factors are not necessarily directly related to the NHS but affect health and healthcare needs. We need to be careful not to widen that gap between rich and poor that we know is already growing in this country and has widened still since the pandemic.

I: Do you have any views on the social contract between medicine and patients? But the social contract also involves the government – something you have already touched upon. Both public and healthcare professionals expect certain things from the government? How do we manage that?

ISH: I feel in some ways that social contract has been broken a little in terms of the way that firstly, the politicians have treated medical professionals and then the NHS. They have consistently and specifically briefed against health professionals in the media which has led to the social contract between medicine and government to have broken in a way that can be problematic because each side is losing trust in the other. It certainly needs rebuilding. As I said earlier, there is no doubt that the NHS needs massive investment. Our workforce needs reinvesting in as do physical structures where hospitals and clinics are crumbling. At the present time, healthcare staff including doctors are really exercised about pay and pensions. Unless this is resolved, this is likely to become an increasingly vital issue that will impact on patient care and exodus of staff which is already happening. If doctors leave the NHS because they feel that they are not being paid appropriately for what they are worth, that will impact on patients and their care which will ultimately impact on the government. The government needs to be valuing staff better, and in my opinion, pay is a part of that. Having said that, the pay actually isn't the whole answer as well, because if you are paid as much as you like but if you are working in terrible working conditions, you are not likely to stay. So a lot of this is about basic respect and feeling valued.

I: What are your views on technology such as telehealth and AI, etc. which often work across disciplines and professions? Do you think that common training across disciplines will be helpful?

SH: I think more interdisciplinary training is a good thing because realistically we work alongside each other in teams complementing each other's skills and experience. And so understanding of what each person does is good but also critical. And there are some examples of good practice. Where I work locally, we do some joint training as well across specialties such as child and adolescent psychiatry trainees. I could go on about underfunding of Child and Adolescent Mental Health Services (CAMHS) and the state of underfunding of services where vulnerable children seem to be struggling. That aside, we have some joint training schemes between paediatricians and mental health practitioners, which is really valuable for both sides as not only that they learn what the other person does but also what the other person cannot do. Our training programmes need to be updated to take into consideration some of these new technologies because at the moment these are not included in training. We need to be looking ahead with our training programmes, not looking back to how we have been doing it for the last 20–30 years. We must look ahead to innovations so that these actually are brought in smoothly in as opposed to playing catch-up. There are certainly huge potential benefits with these new ways of working, particularly because there has been an increased interest in how we move more healthcare outside of the hospital settings to where our patients are, which regrettably has not got off the ground. I think there are some good examples. Some integrated care pathways in London that I'm aware of may help in this direction. New technologies will help with that. I think these innovative strategies will benefit patients so that we may not need them to come to the hospitals and certain assessments can be conducted online. There are some crazy statistics about the amount of road traffic as a direct result of people travelling to and from NHS appointments. It is a lot larger than I had appreciated. So it would be good for the patient but it will also be very good for the environment as well to actually improve that.

I: That's very interesting because I hadn't thought of the pressures on transport and environment till you mentioned it just now.

SH: Recently as I was writing something the figures came to me. It is really quite a high proportion of road traffic and much more than you'd expect. So that is another benefit.

I: Is there anything else that you would like to raise that we have not covered?

SH: Nothing else that comes to mind.

I: Thank you so very much. I really enjoyed talking to you.

SH: Thank you for letting me get on my soapbox.

6 Sir David Haslam

Sir David Haslam is a writer and healthcare policy consultant and a past Chair of the National Institute for Health and Care Excellence (NICE). He is a former President and Chairman of Council of the Royal College of General Practitioners, past-president of the British Medical Association and is Professor of General Practice at the University of Nicosia. He was a GP in Cambridgeshire for 36 years and was Visiting Professor in Primary Health Care at de Montfort University, Leicester, an expert member of the NHS National Quality Board, and National Clinical Adviser to both the Care Quality Commission and the Healthcare Commission. He has written 14 books, mainly on health topics for the lay public and translated into 13 languages, and well over 2,000 articles for the medical and lay press. He was awarded CBE in 2004 for services to medicine and healthcare and was knighted in 2018 for services to NHS leadership.

Interview

I: Thanks very much David for agreeing to be interviewed. You have been in incredibly powerful positions over your career. Over that time how do you think the NHS has functioned or not functioned? What do you see as its strengths and its weaknesses?

DH: I think the NHS is one of the great developments of humankind. It reflects the ability of a society to provide healthcare for its citizens irrespective of their wealth, irrespective of their standing in society. A couple of years ago I had cancer myself and after I'd had my first course of radiotherapy I recall saying to myself, "Isn't it astonishing to live in a country where my fellow citizens have just paid for and provided that care, in the same way that I've paid for and provided for their care?". For me, it is a real mark of a civilised society. That certainly doesn't mean that there are no problems with the National Health Service.

In terms of its aspiration and its vision, it is something of fundamental importance. Its immense strength is its universality. The fact

DOI: 10.4324/9781003382188-6

that it is there for everyone. Of course, as with almost everything in life, the flip side of being universal for the entire population with no clear delineation of what its aspirations means that potentially there is infinite demand, and allied with an inevitably finite resource, the NHS is always going to be under pressure.

In addition, what requires treatment today would not have been seen that way a hundred years ago. A while ago, I read the biography of a general practitioner practising in the 1880s. Almost everything that doctor was seeing in clinical practice, we have now wiped out and yet despite this we are busier than ever. And if you extrapolate that forward and I see no reason why that shouldn't be the case 100 years from now. This presents a real dilemma of constantly changing aspirations, but inevitably finite resource. And the final weakness is that the NHS has developed either intentionally or unintentionally, a sort of benign paternalism, which I think many clinicians and patients have enjoyed. That paternalism is no longer appropriate. There needs to be much more of a partnership between doctors, other clinicians and patients than there was in the past.

I: As you say the NHS is universal and demand is infinite. As you were involved in NICE there was always pressure to approve new and expensive drugs and assess their role in clinical outcomes. And, as you know, there has always been this debate about what kind of treatment and what are the potential outcomes and value for money. So how do we square that circle?

DH: There are two real sources of demand. One is entirely reasonable patient expectations, hopes and aspirations. And the other is the developments produced by the pharmaceutical industry. I certainly don't see the pharmaceutical industry in negative terms, but all too often they develop products and then search for a use for them. Your speciality is an intriguing one. For example, the concept of shyness as being something that requires a selective serotonin reuptake inhibitor is fascinating. I could probably argue for both sides of that debate. But there is a real problem in that we aspire to the World Health Organisation definition of health, i.e. a state of perfect physical and mental and social well-being, rather than simply the absence of illness. That's not something I've ever had, other than fleetingly. You've probably never had that either. So what is it? What is the point that we're trying to achieve in maintaining health? When do we say no? One of the problems for me is that the new and exciting always seems to trump the old and trusted. A new cancer drug at immense expense which offers a tiny advantage but a provably cost-effective advantage over another cancer drug, will tend to get supported and funded. On the other hand, supporting primary care to deliver continuity of care which has been demonstrated to have a far greater benefit on patient health tends to be ignored. It would be nice to have those resources. This fascinates me and this applies to healthcare systems across the world. The technically new and exciting gets politicians excited and gets funded, whereas the seemingly boring things like continuity, relationships, care and humanity which do benefit the patients and affect outcomes tend to get ignored and left behind.

I: You would have seen in your practice that very often patients will bring printouts from the net asking for specific drugs or interventions whether they work or not so how do we manage patients' rights versus responsibilities? So on the one hand it is patients' rights and responsibilities and on the other our expectations of patients and their responses as clinicians?

DH: It is interesting because I think many of us over the last decades have been increasingly vocal about the importance of medicine being done with patients rather than to them. It should be a partnership between the doctor and the patient. Whose body is it anyway? I feel that there is an imbalance of knowledge and experience, and that imbalance works in both directions. Of course, the patient with diabetes has diabetes 24 hours a day, 365 days a year. They know much more about the experience of diabetes than the doctor they see occasionally. And yet the scientific knowledge is not balanced in the same way. Working out the balance between those two things is intriguing. And there isn't a simple answer to it.

We cannot and should not simply go back to the days of when doctors knew best, things are done to the patient, and patients should simply be happy to get what they were given. We couldn't do that anyway. Media publicity for drugs that may or may not be helpful, and issues such as direct-to-consumer advertising in the States all generate increasing cost. Society has to recognise that this constant escalation of expectation cannot continue unchecked, which is why I am really pleased that you are doing this work. Society has to decide what it expects and hopes that its health service can deliver.

There may even be aspects of care that can best be delivered by private medicine. For example, if a patient wants a hugely expensive drug, that carries no discernible benefits over another less expensive treatment at their own cost, provided it is safe, then that's probably down to a commercial transaction with the doctor as long as the doctor is honest and open about risks, benefits, side effects, etc. But if a treatment is to be funded by the National Health Service, I don't think it can be as straightforward as a demand-led service. This is a really difficult balance. I talked earlier about paternalism. And for me, it is something I've talked about many times in lectures and presentations. Years ago, I had an American Air Force base next to my practice area, and as a result, I was consulted by quite a lot of the families of American service personnel. I noticed that if I gave them a prescription, they would inevitably have a series of questions about the effect, side effects, duration, working mechanism of the drugs, etc. If I offered the same prescription to the typical British patient, very few questions are asked. They simply said, "Thank you, doctor". This is obviously a much easier way to practice, but it's not healthy.

There are questions which need addressing around the world. Honest, open, patient-centred conversations are critical. A classic example for me revolves around the use of drugs like statins, which undoubtedly are beneficial and justifiable from a cost-effective population perspective. However, talking to my non-medical friends who have been prescribed statins, their view is a simple binary one. Are these drugs helpful or not? And the answer is much more complex than they realise. In NICE, we developed a patient decision aid to try and help patients understand some of the statistics behind this. They would frequently look at the statistics and realise that if a drug is going to, for instance, benefit only 4 patients out of 100, they may well then choose not to take any. But because of the speed at which doctors often have to practise both in primary and secondary care, pressures on time not being able to explain properly and both sides taking things at face value means that we have reached a fairly unsustainable position with many therapies.

I: That takes us neatly into the question of medicine's social contract. The implicit contract between doctors in this case and patients and the government on both sides, can we and if so how do we deliver it?

DH: Particularly in your speciality, it is the challenge of the availability or desirability of drug treatments and talking therapies. Recognition that talking therapy is not available without a waiting list that's so long that the treatment might as well not exist may push clinicians towards drug prescription, but in the long time this is neither desirable nor logical. Frequently these things come down to workforce levels. The under-investment in the National Health Service workforce has been a major problem in the last few decades.

I: I agree. We simply cannot carry on working the way we did 50 years ago.

DH: No.

I: How do we bring in other grades like physician associates and specialist nurses or the pharmacists on board in a much more integrated way than we have done so far? And what do we need to do about their training?

DH: I am absolutely certain that in 50 years we'll look back on the way we practice at present with a degree of astonishment. We will also look back at some aspects of medical education with a degree of mystification. While I understand the potential theoretical benefits of a pathologist or a psychiatrist studying everything at medical school to an equal extent, many of us actually reached a degree of specialisation earlier in our career and could have a much more focused approach.

However, one thing I'm passionate about is the need for generalists both in primary and secondary care. Clinical generalism is a special skill in itself, and one that is undervalued. It is curious and illogical that in medicine the smaller the area of a doctor's expertise, the higher is the prestige rather than actual importance to patients. This is particularly important for patients with multiple complex co-morbidities who require the breadth of a doctor or clinician for clinical management.

In terms of the other clinical professions, it is extraordinary that so much prescribing and the examination of side effects, drug interactions and so on is not handled by the pharmacist who has potentially the most knowledge on the subject in the team. There is a lot that we could do differently. But this also requires the support and understanding of the public so that they do not feel that they are being fobbed off if they don't get to see a doctor. In many general practices, particularly exacerbated by demand and workforce problems, the receptionists will screen and depending upon the initial presenting problem may direct the patient on to an appropriate person in the team such as the physiotherapist or nurse or doctor or others. In such cases, sadly many traditional patients feel fobbed off and let down. They feel that they haven't had their rights if they're not seeing a doctor, and they will complain about that. I find that unsustainable as well. We need to rethink the role of the whole team and that includes the patient who is actually part of the team.

I: if you had the power to redesign the NHS, how would you do it and what would be different?

DH: That is such a huge question. I would start with the basic first principle of universality. I really do believe in that. Talking about alternative funding systems has the potential for widening health inequalities and rarely saves money. It just shifts it to a different pocket that you have to take it out of. But it is still the same money. So I don't want to go for a different funding method.

I would like greater clarity about the actual point of the health services. What is it trying to do? It seems a very simple question, but I have yet to find an answer to the question even though I have talked to health ministers around the globe. Typically, they look at me as if I'm completely crazy for asking it. We need a clear answer and understanding so that the function is clear. I would involve citizens' juries rather than any other methodology. Society has to take on board this imbalance between infinite demand and finite resource. This has to be addressed somehow and somewhere. I don't think that is simply for the medical profession to discuss. Society should think about this and work with the clinical professions. Back in 2002, George Alberti and Chris Ham wrote a wonderful paper in the BMJ about what they called the social compact between government, doctors and patients and how that has broken down, and we need to relook at that. I was re-reading it recently and not a word of it is out of date.

In the last couple of days, we have had the prime minister standing on a Conservative Party conference stage promising all sorts of things for the health service in terms of reducing waiting times and so on that are completely unachievable. This driving up demand without resource is something that cannot continue, and I am sure society recognises that. In any redesign, we need absolute focus on workforce delivery, which is going to require quite a lot of re-engineering. Who do we need? We have a curiously and bizarrely old-fashioned model of the clinical teams, which really hasn't changed much since 1948 in terms of primary care and secondary care. There have been lots of shifts, nurse practitioners and extended roles of certain clinicians and the development of paramedics in taking on all sorts of roles both in primary and community care. But we haven't really done it from the needs perspective because we have not done the needs analysis. We need to do that and then try to decide what resources are required to help that population. I also find the restrictions on medical school numbers driven by the Treasury quite bizarre and unacceptable. I understand that there have to be limits, but there are major ethical questions in constantly recruiting from overseas, frequently from countries that have greater need than we do. I would like to look at workforce needs and numbers. I would also like to see what we are trying to achieve. I want to look at the boundaries of healthcare as well as the reality of patient and societal expectations.

I: You mentioned the limits of healthcare and what healthcare can and cannot do. What about the models that we have in division between primary, secondary and tertiary care and integration or lack thereof between social services, public health, mental health?

DH: The division is entirely arbitrary. Sometimes I think that the way we have subdivided health issues is a bit like the way the European nations subdivided Africa in the colonial era. Based on absolutely no logic but just drawing lines everywhere. We have a lot of specialism focused around the interests of the doctor rather than the needs of the patients. There are more people in UK society with two or more long-term conditions than there are with one long-term condition. And yet the design of many hospital departments assumes that you have one condition. An example that I have talked about in the past is the research into rheumatoid arthritis suggests that the things that matter most to patients are issues like tiredness and depression, which are very much part of the syndrome. However, all too often they are told by a specialist rheumatologist, that they are unable to help these symptoms and need to see a GP or mental health team. It fascinates me that in this example the concern that matters most to the patient is the thing that really doesn't interest the doctor. To me that seems a very odd way of designing a service. I would like much more to look at the best way of helping real patients rather than theoretical patients based on divisions into specialties, which may have been appropriate in 1948.

I: I have been very interested in distinction between disease and illness in psychiatry. We are trained to deal with diseases, whereas patients are much more interested in illness. I find that they can live with their symptoms as long as they have money, relationships, food, employment, etc. As you say, often the clinicians say this is nothing to do with me. We see them for short periods even if it is frequent we have little idea of what they are doing rest of the time. As you said patient with diabetes has diabetes 365 days a year and we see them for short periods only. With the advent of the apps or smart-watches we can understand deterioration in symptoms. But medical students sometimes have said that they did not come into medicine to become technicians. Technology is important in helping us in understanding, investigating and managing illnesses but how do we bring that together in a humanistic way of training and teaching?

DH: I have got absolutely no evidence for this theory at all but that does not stop me talking about it. For a long time I have thought that all too often we choose the wrong people to become doctors. Partly because we base it on grades with the highest possible A-level results plus grade eight in several musical instruments and to have worked in a care and just astonishing levels of achievement. And most of those A-levels will be in science, in pure sciences, physics, chemistry, biology, maths, all of which are subjects that generally have correct answers. Then we put them into a profession which is packed with uncertainty, especially in mental health and general practice, and then we wonder why they struggle. I am pretty sure that if we selected from a group of people who were adequately bright but had a broader understanding of human nature this would benefit both the doctors and their patients. I have never once knowingly used any of the biochemistry I learnt as a student, but an understanding of the novels of Dickens or Thomas Hardy and the human relationships in those may well be of far more value to the reality in the sort of medicine that is practised now. I am really keen that there should be doctors who are absolute experts at understanding the complexity of biochemistry and Krebs Cycle and all the rest. But that's not the case for many doctors and I think we choose the wrong people, then put them in the wrong jobs and then wonder why they burn out. As I said, I have got no academic evidence to back that theory at all, it is an observation. I also know that some of the best doctors I know happened to get the worst A-level results. Fascinating.

I: I think you're absolutely spot on. Over the years I have come across people who are aware of the arts and culture tend to be much more empathic and able to work with the patient at the level that the patient is able to deal with. So there's an almost equitable relationship. In addition, I think they are also much better being able to deal with uncertainty and ambiguity which are often found in medicine, in some branches more than others. In terms of training, how do we bring physical, mental, public health together? One of the things that has frustrated me in psychiatry has been that we teach psychiatry far too late in medical school. Ideally I would like to start it from day 1. So that patients are assessed and managed in a complete and holistic way. So how do we do that?

DH: The logical question is the exact opposite one. Why wouldn't you? We are talking about real patients. We are not talking about Islets of Langerhans dysfunction. We are talking about people suffering from whatever the condition is. Of course, scientific research is demonstrating that the body-mind split is becoming less and less relevant. The impact of physical inflammation on mental health and mental health issues on the development of other conditions seems to me to be becoming more and more clear. That is why when I said the way we split up conditions has been pretty arbitrary and somewhere in the future we will question the rationale for the split and too frequent referring of patients on to a specialist which brings us back to super-specialisation.

I: Do you think there is any mileage in having some common training between medical students and occupational therapists and nurses and physician associates so that you start off with some common understanding of what each discipline does, and which may also help develop some kind of team spirit.

DH: Yes, probably. It would have to be done very carefully because the tendency of tribes to develop in the clinical world is quite extraordinary. I remember watching young doctors start work in general practice and start talking about "bloody hospital doctors", and then they go and do a job in hospital and start talking about "bloody GP's," whilst everybody complains about the managers. It cannot go on like that. It has to be much more working together. And yes, I think joint training and joint understanding and joint recognition of each other's skills really matter. Like you, I trained a long time ago so I am not really in a position to comment on what's actually happening on the ground now. But I have been astonished how little doctors know about the professions allied to medicine. And yet they're still quite happy to tell them what to do. It seems completely bizarre.

I: You talked earlier about funding models and workforce planning. How do we make it happen?

DH: It's difficult to answer that. My immediate reaction is to look at how the other industries cope with this. And whilst there are differences in healthcare, I'm sure there's expertise in determining workforce needs that we could listen to. It is not the same as bringing in a boss of a supermarket and asking them to reorganise the health service. For me, it is identifying and analysing the needs and then balancing the needs and what is deliverable and what's affordable. One of the major difficulties is the timespan between someone going into medical school and coming out at the other end as a generalist or a specialist by which time the needs of society may well have changed. So I think we need to look at the needs and training which matches those needs. We need clinicians but also those who work with stem cells. When I talk to young doctors now, I say to them that by the end of their career they will be going to be doing stuff that doesn't currently exist. So I can't advise you on that but what is needed is an ability to learn to adapt. That flexibility is absolutely the key for a career in medicine.

I: Bearing in mind that you've already said quite clearly that universality is the key, how do we make sure that we get the resources we need?

DH: The critical word in that question is need, isn't it? That then leads to the debate between needs and wants. And that's a really difficult one. And as I said earlier, it is one that would want a citizen's jury to look into. There are probably three key parameters for how we look at care delivery – quality, affordability and access, but it is often difficult to have all three. So if one wants quality and affordability, access may be a problem – waiting lists. High quality and ease of access may well be unaffordable. Rapid access and affordability may lead to poor quality. For instance, in theory, everybody could see their GP tomorrow if the consultations lasted a very short time, but they would not be worth having. Hence, we are constantly titrating that trilemma of issues. We have to find a way through that. It has been done in the past by managing waiting lists. They have got out of control at the moment, largely driven by austerity prior to the pandemic. Certainly the pandemic didn't help but I don't accept that it is the underlying cause of much of what we're facing. Most of the problems we are facing pre-date the pandemic.

I: Often we do not know where the money allocated to the NHS is distributed. People ought to know that of every pound going in, staff costs are x pence. So in a way people need to know where their contributions are going?

DH: There is a difference with healthcare. That is to do with the balance of knowledge. I do think people have not the least idea what healthcare costs really are. We certainly saw at the time of the Blair and Brown governments what the impact of extra resource could be on waiting times and quality. But money isn't automatically the answer to everything. If you look at the United States they are pouring money into a system which does not guarantee quality. Clarity and justice is what we should be aiming for. So many of these approaches to healthcare become complex because that has to fit in with fundamental philosophical views on life and justice. Some of the most interesting work is by a friend of mine from Dartford in the States, a physician called Al Mulley, who was at the King's Fund and did some work on what he calls "preference, misdiagnosis". His observation that doctors are terribly bad at judging the preferences of their patients, as exemplified by the intriguing fact that doctors tend to choose less treatment for themselves for a given condition than they offer to their patients. To me, that seems like a source of immense potential waste, which is all tied up with not engaging the patient and explaining to them taking a paternalistic approach saying that we're going to do this to you rather than exploring options with patients. It is becoming a cliché, but exploring what matters to the patient as well as what's the matter with them should be the cornerstone of practice. I know that a lot of people who have joint replacements are disappointed. They did not understand what it was that they'd be able to do after the joint replacement. Similarly often there is an assumption that women with particular breast diseases will want a mastectomy rather than a lumpectomy. That choice must be fully explored with the patient. I think that's a really important area that can make a real difference to the healthcare.

I: Have you come across a model that you think we ought to look at more closely and seriously? Particularly funding?

DH: I have not seen a model that makes me say "I would like that one", but there are bits of various models that I admire enormously. I admire Cuba's approach to care like maternal health and child health, because they are a very poor country. Clinicians are very low paid and yet they have the lowest maternal mortality figures – so much better than the United States, who pay much more. I am not recommending that we take on the Cuban system, but they have put a real focus on primary care and on preventive medicine. In this country, we tend to do the opposite. Over the last decade, the proportion of funding going into primary care has gone down. Every Secretary of State for health talks about the importance of prevention and then cuts the budget. Both the World Health Organization and the World Bank have recommended investment in primary care but the budget keeps getting cut. I think that's probably because of shroud waving from some of the secondary care specialties.

Care in part of the United States can be fantastic especially if you are rich and well insured and probably the best in the world. But for the vast majority of the population, it is much worse than much of the world. In theory, many health maintenance organisations (HMOs) have a good system delivering care for a population. It doesn't quite apply to the United Kingdom because many HMOs exclude certain groups from their care model. And, of course, my number one principle is universality and the need to address health inequalities. The more equal a society is, the happier it is. I would dearly like our society to be happier, content and finally rid of the inequalities. It is very clear that if you really want good health outcomes, it's not just health that you invest in but also education and employment, along with investment in infrastructure, elimination of poverty, overcrowding, and so on. One can't just keep pouring money into healthcare while still letting diets deteriorate and social interaction to worsen.

I: Health rather tragically often has been seen in isolation as a silo. But as you say we must invest in education, housing and employment and a whole range of ministries ought to be working together.

DH: Yes. Absolutely right. I mean, I love the quote by Desmond Tutu, that if you see drowning people flowing past you in a stream, you can leap in and keep pulling them out. Or you can go upstream and see why they are falling in in the first place. And our system does not do that. It puts all the effort and all the energy into pulling people out of the stream when they're in crisis. I understand the politics of that from a political perspective. We see that exciting news stories focusing on the treatment of individual patients with names will always trump reports about prevention or better outcomes for a population because in the latter there is no one identifiable to write about. Stories about the treatment of heart attacks are naturally seen as far more interesting and exciting than a report about heart attacks that didn't happen because of preventative interventions. I am absolutely not saying that we ought to stop funding medical specialties. But there is no doubt that the balance of funding at present is wildly out of kilter for where the benefit could be greatest.

I: Thanks very much David. Really appreciate your time.

7   Dr Richard Horton

Dr Richard Horton is editor-in-chief of *The Lancet*, a United Kingdom-based medical journal. He is an honorary professor at the London School of Hygiene and Tropical Medicine, University College London and the University of Oslo. He studied medicine at University of Birmingham, England, and then worked at the Liver Unit in Royal Free Hospital. In 1990, he became assistant editor of *The Lancet* and five years later became its editor-in-chief in the United Kingdom. He has advised the WHO and the United Nations on a number of issues related to clinical trials, refugees and health matters. He has published widely. He wrote *Second Opinion*, a book with his collected writings and has recently produced a volume on Covid. He is a powerful advocate for issues affecting medicine and has been honoured widely.

Interview

I: Thanks very much for sparing the time, great to see you. I did send the list of questions but many of them will have overlapping responses so we may not need to go through all. If we start by looking at your perceptions on the current state of the NHS?

RH: I am going to speak as a user of the National Health Service as well as an observer of the NHS. For the past 3–4 years, I've had the pleasure of being a frequent attender of hospitals in the NHS. And despite the enormous scrutiny and often criticism that the NHS receives in the political and public spheres, my personal view is that we do have a simply superb national health service that delivers certainly extremely high-quality care for the majority of patients. Now, that's not to say that there are no weaknesses. The common complaint is that the NHS is only good for acute care, but for chronic care it tends to fall down. I think that generalisation goes too far. My overall score for the NHS is that it's doing remarkably well under extreme challenges and difficult circumstances and in the face of ever-growing demand.

DOI: 10.4324/9781003382188-7

I: Almost everyone interviewed for this book agrees that acute care in the NHS is absolutely superb but it falls for people with multiple chronic co-morbid conditions. There is a resulting tension between hospital and community and social care. Do you see that as an issue?

RH: I don't think that the current model of primary care in the community and secondary care or tertiary care and hospitals works well today. I think that's a model that was successful at the birth of the National Health Service and worked reasonably well for several decades. However, we have now reached a level of complexity of healthcare which means that the general practitioner simply cannot give a credible advice to a patient for many of the most complex health conditions that they may be suffering from. The therapeutic advances that have taken place in medicine mean that a GP just is not a credible interlocutor to sit between the hospital and the patients. So for many patients with chronic disease, now it is the hospital which is the primary care centre. Hence you have to ask, whether that is a sensible model? And the answer is of course it is not. What we currently have is that the hospital has evolved into the primary care setting for many patients – the principal points at which they intersect with the health system. We have not created a decentralised system outside the hospital where one can access specialists. By specialists I don't just mean hospital specialists, I mean specialist generalists who can deal with a patient in a community setting. I think the workforce structure we have is not fit for purpose and the institutional structure is also not fit for purpose. We're basically trying to run a 21st century healthcare service with a 20th century health system, and that is simply not sustainable. This will unfortunately lead to continuing erosion in the quality of care.

I: Assuming the NHS did not exist and you had the power to set up and design it on a blank sheet of paper, what would you do in this current social context?

RH: We clearly need hospitals as centres for advanced surgical diagnostic medical care. But we also need services for the long-term management of many conditions. If you look at the bulk of morbidity is around the cardiovascular disease, cancer, metabolic disease and mental ill -health. My question is: is the general practitioner sufficiently well trained to deal with the complexities of modern management of those conditions particularly complex co-morbidities? And the clear answer is that they are not. There is no way that a general practitioner can be familiar with the intricacies of the complications of multiple immunotherapies for different cancers, as well as the complexities of managing heart failure in a patient with other co-morbidities, let alone trying to manage a patient with major depressive disorder. In order to span all of those management issues and be a credible mediator between hospital and community. It is an expectation that cannot be fulfilled. I would devolve chronic care into the community, not in general practices as we currently have them. I would set these up in a network of polyclinics where you have generalists who are trained in specialist areas. For example, we would have a group of generalists who had special training in cardiovascular disease, or cancers, or respiratory disease, infectious diseases or mental health creating a network of specialist generalists. Based in the community, they will be better able to manage complex co-morbid conditions. I am not saying that from an abstract theoretical perspective. I say this as somebody who's been using the health service for a chronic condition for the past 3–4 years and have seen the absurd way in which we manage complex health conditions. As I said earlier, this has turned the hospitals into primary care centres and existing primary care centres have been completely disintermediated and cut out of the loop of specialist care simply because doctors there don't have the necessary skills to manage them. This pressure on the system is only going to grow in the future. So why are we not able to change it? The problem is not political. It is professional. We have a set of professional tribes in medicine that have so many vested interests to defend that you will simply not see general practice, which is treated more as a religion than a specialty, give up its so-called rights of generalist community care. Equally hospital specialists who enjoy their privileged position and palaces of medical power do not want to see themselves devolved into the community settings. And while we have our existing system of Royal Colleges as professional organisations defending the status quo, we are not going to see any progress at all. One of the challenges is professional, but it is also tribal. If I were to speak with the President of a Royal College of Physicians and proposed that consultants need to go out of hospitals into the community working side by side with general practitioners, there would be a collective intake of breath. They are likely to go into supraventricular tachycardia because that would be an anathema to a physician. But similarly, if you said to general practitioners that they needed further training to learn more about the nature of modern therapeutics in a particular domain of medicine, for an additional period, again you'd be regarded as somehow an apostate. You were somehow going against the biblical tradition of general practice, which probably has these quasi-religious connotations. You have to believe in general practice and its philosophy. And if you don't believe in it, then you need to be struck out of the community. For a profession that's supposed to be based on science, we are remarkably narrow minded and anti-scientific in the way that we think about the design of the health service.

I: Having community polyclinic centres does not appear to be dissimilar from the cottage hospitals that existed?

RH: No, it's not. The town in the West country that I grew up in had a cottage hospital which had GPs as the attending physicians on a rotating basis. And the specialists from the hospital would come and visit patients from time to time. I am talking about a proper centre. For example, a patient with cancer who has had immunotherapy in the hospital and these numbers are on the increase, surely they can be followed up by specialists in the community. There is not much point in following them up at the hospital and yet that's where they are followed up. Now, the general practitioner can't follow them up because they may not have a clue about immunotherapy, its complications, etc. I am not being mean or insulting, but the simple fact is that there will also be very many other conditions where the GP may have some generalised knowledge but not a specialist one. It's just the fact that various fields in medicine are moving so fast that it's just not possible for generalists to keep up in this way. So it would be better that these patients are seen in the community by specialists so that hospitals are not under pressure. They should be seen by doctors who have a generalist basis for the specialist interest. And unfortunately, we're not training those kinds of doctors. So that's what I mean by centres which are a slightly different model.

I: I understand what you are saying. We need both specialists and generalists but most people want to specialise because it gives them status. Let's take the example of an orthopaedic surgeon who only operates on the left hand. Now that is incredibly important. And I have always thought that we need generalists, but we also need specialists, as you say, that some generalists could do some speciality training in a particular field, so they are both generalists and specialists. But this specialism can go really extreme. Specialists also need to have some basic generalist knowledge and awareness.

RH: That's absolutely true. Of course, there is always going to be a need for specialists and even super-specialists but a specialist surgeon is not going to be spending half his or her time in the community at a polyclinic. You do need to have a group of people who are doing ultra- specialist work, and that's going to require being in a tertiary or secondary care setting. If I wake up feeling unwell and am not sure what is wrong with me, seeing a generalist will be quite useful. I would also question whether that generalist needs to be a doctor. During triage and also entry into the healthcare system, do we really need a medically qualified person? Our profession tells us that we do need 5–6 years of training because the world is incredibly complex and we should not cut corners. You and I both know that's complete nonsense. If there is someone who is fully trained in recognising presentation of certain symptoms, making a differential diagnosis, then they can guide the person, but equally importantly, if they are uncertain, then they can refer them to perhaps a generalist doctor. It is certainly possible to have physician assistants, nurse practitioners, and others have a much greater role in the health service. It always surprises me that we do not use skills of pharmacists as much as we could. In many countries around the world, pharmacists play a key role in the health system. Instead we train and use pharmacists to be business managers in the local chemists which is utterly ridiculous. We can do a lot more with allied health professionals, which is such a derogatory term. It is clear to me that other health professions could play a much greater role as access points to the health system. Individuals could then see their general practitioners if needed, some of whom may stay more generalist. A large number of healthcare professionals could then get a degree of specialist training so that they can manage cases in the community. This then frees up the hospitals which can have the super-specialists dealing with complex cases which may need more sophisticated investigations and interventions. However, in order to do that requires a willingness of the profession to change. Tragically, what we have seen over the decades is that our profession does not want to change because you used the word status. There appears to be an inbuilt status anxiety attached to change within the professions.

I: As you know we are trained in silos. After finishing medical school and specialist training which are by and large in silos doctors are expected to work in teams and even lead them. So individuals have to change their mindset. I am very interested in your views if there is any mileage in having a period of common learning across disciplines to spend a few months together to get to know what each other does.

RH: I completely agree. This notion of inter-professionalism, into professional training, needs to be at the heart of the future of professional education. And again, it comes back to status and hierarchy. There is a hierarchy of health professions, which unfortunately, we aid and abet in medicine. Imagine going to medical school and spending not your first three months, but your first year with lectures or seminars or tutorials or ward work or community work side by side with nurses, pharmacists and others. I think that would build a respect for the members of the health team that you would eventually become part of. Unfortunately that simply doesn't exist today. Even now medical students are not taught that. Since our training there has been no solution in the way we educate young doctors. Actually that is pretty shocking. The fact is that we do not teach the basics about the multi-professional team that is now required to manage patients. We imagine that after the foundation years, the doctor will somehow magically be able to fit into a team and understand the roles of other members of the team. Of course, it is nonsense. But again, where is the leadership from us and our profession? There is absolutely no leadership.

I: We touched upon hospital care and community care, then there is social care, but also potential for integration between mental health and physical health. And then public health is somewhere out there which due to defunding of local councils is becoming even less of a priority. So how do we bring it all together? I see working together of physical health and mental health, as quite a big challenge. We as psychiatrists are often not confident enough to deal with physical problems and often physicians do not feel very comfortable dealing with psychiatric problems. Where did we go wrong and what we do about it?

RH: Well, we can blame Descartes. It is very interesting. It was some years ago now we published some work from the Deep End Projects General Practice Project in Scotland, which looked at basically three coordinates: physical health, mental health and social deprivation. Looking at it, it is clear that physical and mental health are tracked together on a social gradient. On seeing that we can also recognise that our health system is simply not evolved to deal with physical and mental health comorbidities which are presenting according to social disparities. Several points emerge from that observation. Firstly we have completely separated the biological from the social and that has been a huge and longstanding mistake. That has been illustrated effectively by the pandemic which was indeed syndemic – a synthesis of epidemics, the biological and the social interactions. These combinations created the risk profile for Covid-19. That is not a new observation. We've known that for so long that it was just concentrated into a short space of time. This separation of the biological and social in teaching and practice of medicine and in the organisation of services in the NHS remains a problem. Secondly, we have marginalised public health to the point where it has almost disappeared today in a country which was the birthplace of public health and social medicine. It is not just a tragedy, it is criminal. Again, we have a public health leadership that is invisible. Equally tragically we have a broader medical community that simply isn't interested in public health. The only jewel in the crown of public health is that we still have a nucleus of a public health research community which is strong, but not very politically or professionally engaged. Thirdly as you are drawing the attention to the artificial division between the psychological and the physical, which reflects our training as we don't teach psychological medicine side by side with physical medicine. If you study cardiology in a clinical attachment, you are not taught to look at the mental health of the patient or even the implications of cardiac problems on mental wellbeing of the patient. You're not taught or trained on the mental health dimensions of physical illnesses whether it is heart disease, cancer or any other physical illness. Similarly psychiatrists often do not look at implications of psychiatric disorders on physical health and wellbeing of their patients. As we have separated these in our education system, tragically this has caused that status anxiety and tribalism that I mentioned earlier. In some ways, it is an inadvertent consequence of unnecessary specialisation. But what we haven't done is then to step back and recognise that there has been an enormous cost as a result of that separation of powers. We need to bring them back together. However, if I went to a professor of cardiology and said, I'd like to introduce a module on the mental health dimensions of living with heart disease, he or she would look at me as if I've gone crazy. From my experience as a user of the health service, it is clear that at times the most pressing need is psychological and not necessarily physical but that is where the physicians focus. There is absolutely nothing provided for you in the psychological domain, even in our most prestigious hospitals. So we have an enormous shortfall in that. It invites you to ask, Dinesh, doesn't it? We are saying all this and we know all this as do our colleagues, but nothing changes. And that is what I find really strange that none of this is radical or unknown or hidden as everybody knows this and has done so for a long time and yet there is major resistance to change. There are reasons why things do not change and understanding and changing that is itself a major challenge.

I: There are several issues related to that. It is that the specialties are under attack from different sources so they tend to retreat into their comfort zones rather than looking at the bigger picture and trying to change things. If I had the power I would push for teaching of psychiatry from day 1 of medical school as well as specialist training. So how do we bang heads together?

RH: Absolutely. No question. Absolutely. Medicine must acknowledge the social aspects of illnesses recognising and dealing with it in causation and management in an integrated way. I feel that part of the reason for reluctance may well be great fear of politicians destroying the fundamental model of the NHS, being free healthcare at the point of demand. Sometimes we worry that if we're critical of the

NHS in public, then we play into the hands of those who want to destroy what we think of such a valuable entity. Also, both of us know that many of our colleagues in senior leadership positions do not want to be critical because they feel that if they are critical, they will lose their seats at the table of government and so they go along. In a recent conversation a President confirmed this by saying exactly that were they critical they would not be invited to the table. If that is the line and position we take and not raise our voices then nothing will change. And we would just see a constant erosion of quality because the system isn't evolving with the needs of the population at the present time along with professionalisation of our tribes into colleges creating tribes and tribalism, which are all about protecting themselves rather than advancing the field more generally. And we've basically a recipe for status.

I: It is a constant battle for funding. On a daily basis, newspapers are full of stories of crises in the NHS which are often blamed on a lack of funding. How do we manage funding?

RH: Of course, money is important because new technologies whether in reaching diagnosis or treatment are expensive, which takes money away from other parts of the NHS budget. So money is of course an important component, but I think we spend too much time talking about money. Money is not the main problem in the NHS. The main problem in the NHS is that we've got a system that's not designed for the needs of the population. And just throwing more money at the NHS to carry on that system without pretty radical reform isn't going to be helpful. Talking about money is too easy. We need to talk much more about the workforce, about the design of the system, about these issues of education, into professionalism and so on. We don't seem ready or prepared to do that.

I: Everybody I have spoken to has raised the issue of workforce and a lack of workforce planning. And as long as I have been in the NHS, it did come as a surprise to me that there's absolutely no workforce planning.

RH: It is incredible, isn't it, that we don't and I don't know enough about the history of why that is. It is not simply about numbers. So Keir Starmer says that he will increase the number of medical students by 6000 but that is not the only point. It is about the fundamental roles of all health professionals. How does a member of the public enter the health system? Currently the barriers are high to get onto a general practice list and go through a receptionist to get to see a doctor. This is a crazy way. When we have such a massive demand for healthcare as we have, to keep our triage system the way we had it in 1948 is just crazy. What other part of society has not changed for 75 years, like our organisation of professionals? It would be unacceptable in any other business, profession or service. But we haven't changed in 75 years because of the power blocs that were created as a result of the social political contract that Bevan made with the profession in 1948 along with the trade-offs that had to be made in order to set up the NHS. Those basic political contracts exist today, and these are dirty and rusty and surrounded by cobwebs, but exist and have not been cleared. We must break and rewrite these but nobody has got the courage to break and change that contract.

I: That goes back to the point of social contract that you and I had talked about before. There is a social contract between medicine and society, including patients and then between society and the government and government and the medical profession. One of the big concerns that has quite often been raised is about the implicit nature of the contract because the contract is implicit. It should not be explicit but it links with patients' rights versus responsibilities. As you said both new interventions, and new investigations are expensive and the demand keeps rising. Also patient expectations have changed too. What are your thoughts on patient rights versus responsibilities?

RH: When we talk about patient responsibilities, we need to be clear. What does that mean? And I'm very nervous about that because the public isn't stupid. They choose to do things often because of the environment which they're in. Can we really say that if somebody is unemployed and they have a chronic health condition it is entirely their fault? They may be living in a community where the schools are terrible, the environment itself is awful and they do not have access to good medical services, is it unreasonable that that person smokes 20 cigarettes a day, drinks a bottle of vodka every couple of days and doesn't do any physical activity. I would say that their reaction to the social conditions is completely normal. If you've got no hope in your life because of the world and the environments around you, then self-destructive or unreasonable behaviours seems perfectly understandable. We could talk about patients' responsibilities in that situation, but it is not very helpful. This is where the government does need to take a role. Also this is where commercial determinants of health are now becoming increasingly important and part of the health agenda. The role of corporate power particularly food in shaping the environment in which we live is of immense importance. It is clear that commercial determinants are significant in that unless we put a constraint on corporate power that shapes our environments and shapes health behaviours, no amount of medicine under these circumstances, or patient responsibilities and patient rights are going to solve that. This epidemic of non-communicable diseases that we face today includes mental and physical health and has to be managed by the government stepping in to regulate some markets, which are extraordinarily damaging for health, otherwise we are in bigger trouble.

I: You touched upon something earlier about setting up services and the way we need to think outside the box. How do you see the role of technology and in mental health, e-health, AI, etc., in the scheme of things?

RH: I think technology has an important part to play in terms of accessing the health system. I've seen for myself the role that telephone appointments, video appointments and online booking of appointments can have. Three years ago, we could not book an online appointment for a blood test. But thanks to the pandemic, now I can book my blood test online at a specific time and on a specific day which is good for me. It should be possible to book an appointment with a health professional in the same way. Such an approach should be possible using technology that would be easy to introduce. I'm much more sceptical about the idea of digital technology solving some of our health challenges. Most digital technologies today are expensive, they're not sustainable and the evidence just isn't there to prove that they've had any demonstrable benefit for patients. I think that the whole discussion about artificial intelligence is enormously hyped. Then there is the question of cost, evidence and sustainability. I am sure it will have an impact. However, fundamentally, medicine is a human discipline. Medicine is about two human beings not only facing each other but listening to each other, trusting each other, and believing in each other and no amount of technology should get in the way of that. There's something irreducible about what medicine is and technology can assist that. But if we ever think hubristic, that technology can replace that human dimension to what medicine is, we make a huge, huge, huge mistake.

I: I couldn't agree more. You're absolutely right. Does the NHS have a future?

RH: The NHS has a very bright future. Because of my personal experience, Dinesh, I am a massive supporter of the National Health Service. I've always used the NHS. I always will use the NHS. I think that it faces existential challenges for the reasons we've discussed. Tribalism amongst the profession, rapidly advancing therapeutics and technological advances in medicine and ossification of the system, a lack of leadership from the profession are some of the challenges that need addressing urgently if the NHS is to survive. There are many problems yet at the heart of medicine and at the heart of the NHS, we have people who are utterly dedicated to what they do. And I have nothing but enormous gratitude and admiration for what they do. They will keep the NHS alive despite the mistakes of everybody else. So I wish the NHS a happy 75th birthday. But I would plead with so-called leaders to have courage and vision and think about its future more than they presently do.

I: That's a perfect ending. Richard, thank you so much for your time and sharing your thoughts and vision.

8　Baroness Molly Meacher

Baroness Molly Meacher is a crossbench peer who has been active in the House of Lords, particularly on issues of mental health and drug reform, and whose expertise in health and social care and involvement with the NHS has included being chair of APPG on Drug Policy; she has been chair of East London Mental Health NHS Foundation Trust. She is currently President of the Haemophilia Society. She has written a number of books on mental health, welfare and poverty. She has been involved in a number of Bills dealing with social and healthcare.

Interview

I: Thanks very much for your time. As mentioned I am putting together interviews with different individuals to look at the state of the NHS as we are coming to its 75th anniversary. Shall we start with your views on the current state of the NHS?

MM: It seems to me that the NHS is in a state of crisis. And the reason for that, presumably, is that the pressures of COVID came to a service that was already underfunded. And this has resulted in this spiral of early retirements, people going on to part-time work and people just leaving the service mid-career, which has generated an unsustainable situation. I don't know what the solution is. I really don't. It seems that the government has no idea what to do about the situation and seems to make irrelevant points. That's how I see it at the present time.

I: What do you see as its strengths and weaknesses?

MM: The NHS was set up to deal with acute episodes. And it has always been extremely good at dealing with those episodes, including mental health episodes but very particularly physical, acute episodes. It wasn't really set up with the chronic mental and physical disabilities and problems in mind. It has struggled throughout its existence to deal with chronic illness and remains really rather inadequate in that direction. This has been made a lot worse, I think, over the last

DOI: 10.4324/9781003382188-8

70 years, with families moving further away. Often there are no family members nearby to pick up the pieces as people become frail or continue to be frailer over many years and people assume they can just turn to the NHS. They turn to primary care, and assume that they will be there to deal with any problem that seems to come along. We have an increasing proportion of greying population. Thus, this is a very different demographic now and family structures and family habits. This has had a massive impact on primary care in particular, but also on Accident & Emergency (A&E). Someone mentioned to me the other day that an individual had turned up at the A&E and all they really needed was a sticking plaster. And if somebody back home had been able to put a plaster on them, they wouldn't have needed to turn up at the A&E. Therefore, there is a massive over-expectation in particular of primary care and A&E, and it just isn't sustainable. The greatest strength of the NHS is the quality that it doesn't matter how poor you are, how rich you are, you will get the same treatment and that is a big strength.

I: A part of the problem has been that social care has been out on a limb and health and social care often have not been talking to each other. And that raises very interesting questions as you were saying about families moving away and more and more people living alone and perhaps feeling lonely which can delay help-seeking. But it also raises questions about patients' rights versus responsibilities and how do we deal with those?

MM: That's right. I think patients' expectations are now extraordinarily high. They seem almost to feel they've got a right to access to a doctor come what may. In other countries, they seem to have other ways of dealing with this type of expectations. Pharmacists play a much bigger role in many countries. They do have deeper training so that they can actually do more than they can actually do in this country. Perhaps people should think of going to a pharmacy in the first instance rather than to a doctor. I don't think patients have the right to a non-urgent appointment with a doctor within two weeks. If it is non-urgent, then perhaps it could be dealt with by somebody else. There is a need for far greater development of local support systems now that families are not available, charities like Mind-run group homes but that requires proper funding. Running groups and drop-in centres for people with chronic mental health problems can help avoid admissions and re-admissions. We need to think outside the box rather in terms of meeting patient expectations. I think the government has a job to do in rolling back those expectations actually, and getting across to people that not only doctors are unbelievably stretched but so are other health professionals. Governments all too often play the role of we're on the side of the patient which is right but they don't help in getting the right balance between patients' rights and responsibilities at all. This is something that ought to be dealt with. The other aspect that can be encouraged is the development of the idea of the expert patient. In East London, in mental health, when we took on community services, there were a lot of patients with chronic physical disabilities. We gave them equipment to do their own blood pressure, blood tests, etc. and they all did a lot of work themselves, instead of community staff doing domiciliary visits. The patients would report in to the team who would then decide whether domiciliary visits were really needed. It was a very efficient way of doing something involving patients with greater patient engagement and satisfaction. That cut down on home visits. Thus there are alternate ways of working. We certainly did it very well in East London. It is possible to do it everywhere and maybe people are doing that.

I: The other thing linked up with community support that you mentioned is social prescribing which has taken off in different parts of the country in a very interesting way.

MM: Yes, absolutely. In East London, we tried to get away from seeing people as patients. We set up football teams, bands, art classes separate from art therapy and we found artists. We had, as it were, social prescribing. We recommended that certain patients joined all these different activities rather than just coming along for their medication and it trumped all those people's wellbeing. They still had their psychosis, but somehow they weren't just simply schizophrenic. They were footballers, art workers, etc. Of course, some did have a problem with voices but somehow the symptoms took much more of a back seat as they developed these tremendous interests and skills. Often their whole day was taken up with their music or sports practice so they were not thinking about their symptoms. That is just one very specific bit of social prescribing. I was absolutely staggered at the benefits of providing extra community based involvement.

I: That is absolutely right in that very often patients can live with their symptoms as long as they have a life, they've got a roof over their head, food, money in their pocket, employment or some occupation.

MM: Indeed this is a much better option than if all they've got to think about is their symptoms. Another slightly different thing but related in a way to social prescribing is referring people to groups. I once ran a group of people with bipolar disorder, and then I would attend ward rounds as I was a social worker then, psychiatrists would see the patient and reduce their medication. It would appear that one could actually reduce symptoms through some of these social responses to sickness.

I: When at the beginning of the pandemic, the prime minister asked for 250,000 volunteers, nearly 750,000 people signed up. Why are we not using that human capital to engage with people who may be isolated, lonely, sitting at home? Partly it is the integration of social care and healthcare, and partly it is about engaging the community in some kind of social contract?

MM: Of course, there are an awful lot of voluntary organisations and to some degree they are doing that sort of work. But volunteers also do need managers, they need organising, they need locations. It is important to redirect government and local authority funding to greater development of community activities to deal with loneliness, to deal with chronic illness, to deal with all sorts of problems that people have which will help take some of the pressure from the NHS. I completely agree that there has to be a different way forward. Again, it is responding to the changing demographic and the splitting up of families and people moving. Something has to take their place. And people think that all of this should be done by the NHS. It seems to me that a bit more investment needs to go into voluntary organisations so that with a bit more imagination that work can be done better. Even though a lot of them are doing some of that work but far more could be done in that direction.

I: What is your view on the integration of physical health and mental health and in public health and healthcare? They are all in separate silos and nobody seems to be talking to each other.

MM: Certainly it feels to me as though healthcare and social care should be absolutely integrated. I can't see how it is helpful at all to have them separate. Obviously, a lot of social care is private and contracted out. I would definitely bring those two together. I have thought about mental health and I am not convinced that it should be under one management in any locality because the needs are quite different. Of course, any human being might have mental and physical problems of one sort or another or a mixture of the two. My main priority would be to bring social and physical care together.

I: Over the years, I have thought about integration of physical and mental health. Initially, I thought that it would be really good because it will destigmatise and people can go to one-stop shops. When it came to funding, it became very clear that mental health trusts generally cope better so there was a danger that money may well be taken away from them.

MM: As you say, that may deal with the problem of stigma to a degree but the key thing is the funding. And if you ringfence the funding then integration could be beneficial.

I: How do we make the NHS fit for purpose? If you were redesigning the NHS, what would you do? Let's assume that it doesn't exist. You now have a completely blank slate.

MM: In my view the basics would be the same. I would build a system that looked at the social and health needs of people in one organisation. I see that the main problems are structures. We do not need super-specialisation for an organisation of this size. As we said earlier, society has changed and we have not developed the services accordingly. We may have done it to some extent in a patchy sort of way. There are a lot of voluntary organisations, but if you are starting from scratch to build around the NHS, a lot of social support systems can be developed which require a response from professional people. I would have all these social support systems built around it, but not necessarily under management, but certainly seen as related to it and absorbing a lot of the demand from people.

I: Do you have any thoughts on funding and workforce planning and what are the potential challenges and solutions?

MM: Often, there is a lot of talk about there being far too many managers in the NHS, whereas my understanding is that we actually spend less as a proportion of the total budget on managers in comparison with other good healthcare system. Having said that, we need to have a very good look at the management structure of the NHS and whether we are actually investing adequately in good management of the service. In terms of funding I can only say what others say that it is a huge challenge as the medication, investigation costs are increasing all the time and it just absorbs ever more money. And of course, we all regard health as our number 1 priority. So really, we should be spending quite a lot more on our NHS. It appears that we do spend about 8% of our GDP on health whereas other countries spend more and some spend far less. At least we're up to that but other Western countries spend more. America's expenditure on healthcare is almost double. So, we could spend a lot more on our NHS, and my belief is that we should. People would welcome it. But a part of that money should go into the less expensive support systems around the edge. I do think that is really important.

I: Do you think the NHS has a future?

MM: Well, I have family members in the NHS primary care and they tell me that they envisage primary care going in the direction of that of dentists. In other words, if you're wealthy, you can get a private doctor, and if you're not wealthy, you'll have a second-grade service. I think that is a major threat, actually. And governments need to take hold of it. And our problem is that, of course, I am now going to be political. A string of Conservative governments obviously welcome more and more privatisation. And so my vision for the future is if we continue to have Conservative governments, we can expect ever-increasing privatisation and a two-tier system. On the other hand, if we have a string of Labour governments, then we will probably have greater funding and hopefully we'll hold on to the equality principle, which is fundamental to the NHS.

I: We talked about rights versus responsibilities. And one of the things that has always interested me is the social contract between medicine and patients and patients and government and government and medicine – a tripartite contract. Do you think there is some mileage in developing that further? And going back to what you were saying that patients understand what the NHS is for and politicians know what they are funding and the healthcare staff know where the money is coming from, and where it is going, and a sense of mutual respect and understanding which are all part of that contract.

MM: I do believe that patients certainly need far greater understanding about the NHS, pressures it is under, its funding and alternative sources of support. My main focus will be on educating the public. That seems to me to be the big gap that people just don't have any understanding at all. And I think all our emphasis on complaint systems drives me crazy. When I look at a GP surgery and find a great notice that if you want to complain ring this number. Yes, there may be reasons to complain but people forget that complaints are incredibly expensive, incredibly time-consuming, and most of them are not actually necessary. There is a major challenge here for education and understanding.

I: I have talked to many politicians and suggested that they use charts to explain where each pound is being spent but so far there has been no interest. There seems to be a reluctance to be upfront about the costs and its impact. Is there any way that we can change that?

MM: You are right. It is just one vast pot of money people are aware of, and often have no idea where it goes. I think to have charts in GP surgeries that would be up there in the waiting rooms about spending would be a very interesting idea. And I think it would help people to understand. That's right. Absolute good idea.

I: You said earlier about working with the pharmacists and working with nurses and increasingly there are nurse specialists and physician assistants, etc. Everybody gets trained in silos and yet we are expected to work in teams. So how do we change that? Is there a way? Have you seen any model which can overcome that barrier and so that we learn from each other and maybe learn together.

MM: Oh, that's a huge question, isn't it? Probably beyond my pay grade, I think. There is no doubt that the people's trainings are very, very different. But then when you start working, you've got to learn what each other contributes, and maybe that's the time to do it once you have got all that basic knowledge that you need for your particular specialism. And then of course, during training, doctors spend years in hospitals doing the job and learning a lot during the training about how to work with nurses and pharmacists and others, aren't they? So it all goes on before they start work, actually.

I: Do you have any examples of good clinical practice?

MM: I suppose my expert patient, the example that I gave already. For me that was a very important way of working, making use of a patient's own time and expertise and using equipment in that direction, rather than sending people around the countryside visiting people's homes when they didn't need to. And the social prescribing in managing mental health, which included prescribing of all sorts of things other than medication, such as football or music. What it meant was that medication is only one of what might help somebody.

I: Is there anything else that you wish to say that I haven't covered?

MM: I think we have, actually.

I: Thank you so very much for your time, really appreciate it.

9   Dr Chaand Nagpaul

Dr Chaand Nagpaul is a senior partner in a general practice in North London where he has practised for 33 years. He was the first ethnic minority chair of the British Medical Association (BMA) Council from 2017 to 2022. Prior to that he chaired the BMA's General Practitioners committee. In these roles, he has represented the breadth of the medical profession across the UK to government and policymakers. He has been lobbying for the NHS to be able to deliver equitable, comprehensive quality care and address health inequalities . He led a major BMA project and report *Caring, Supportive, Collaborative*[1] in 2019 which promoted a vision of a health service that is compassionate and supportive of its workforce, with a culture of learning rather than blame and rooted in collaboration between doctors and staff in general practice, the community and hospitals.

Interview

I: Thanks very much Chaand. It will be a free-flowing discussion and we'll pull things together. You have been a general practitioner and having been in the top position in the BMA you are back being a clinician. Just to emphasise that these are your personal views and not of the BMA. So, if that is ok, shall we start?

CN: Yes, of course.

I: What's your view of the NHS at the present time and what are its challenges and weaknesses?

CN: At the present time, there is no doubt that we have a healthcare system in which the demand on the system far exceeds its capacity to deliver. This is having a consequence on the quality and accessibility of care for patients. It relates to all sectors from primary care (including general practice), community services as well as secondary care (hospitals and specialist services). I would categorise capacity both in terms of workforce, that's human resources, but also the infrastructure- these are inadequate to meet the needs of

DOI: 10.4324/9781003382188-9

the population as a result of historic lack of funding. Infrastructure includes hospital beds, equipment as well as estate and IT. We have amongst the lowest numbers of doctors per capita compared to equivalent nations - around 50,000 fewer doctors compared to the OECD average. We also have a live problem of recruitment and retention. There are over 100,000 unfilled vacancies in the NHS, of which about 8000 are doctor posts, and increasing numbers of medics are retiring early or moving abroad. We have about half the numbers of hospital beds compared to OECD averages - Germany for example has 3x as many beds per thousand patients. We have amongst the lowest numbers of diagnostic equipment like MRI and CT scanners per head in Europe, and many GP practices don't have space to meet the needs of increasing levels of care in the community. This is resulting in backlogs of care and low morale on staff affecting recruitment and retention. Setting up a vicious cycle. These pressures are compounded by growing demand for healthcare from people living longer with increased illness, long term conditions and multiple morbidity.

We also have an ethnically diverse workforce where more than one third of doctors have come from abroad, and over four in 10 are from ethnic minority backgrounds. There is evidence of race discrimination in medicine, with doctors from ethnic minorities reporting twice the level of bullying, increased disciplinary procedures, poorer career progression and an ethnicity pay gap. This is preventing ethnic minority doctors from achieving their full potential, which in turn is not allowing the NHS to make full use of the talent of its workforce, in which patients lose out. Worryingly, a recent BMA survey shows that 9% of ethnic minority doctors have left the NHS due to experiences of racism, 23% are considering doing so, and 60% have been off work with sickness or stress. This is inevitably adding pressure to an NHS already suffering from shortages of doctors. It is vital that the NHS is driven by values of equality and inclusivity for its workforce which is vital for recruitment and retention and which needs to be a priority for government cascaded through all NHS leaders in the system.

The NHS has also been afflicted by a negative blame culture, where healthcare professionals often feel unable to speak out, or face recrimination if they do so. This was a key finding from the Francis report on Mid-Staffs but unfortunately 10 years on we are still seeing headlines of major patient safety incidents occurring in the NHS, on a climate of staff afraid to speak out. So when there is a significant event in any hospital the entire system can end up focusing on individuals and detracting from the responsibility of the hospital's senior leadership who are often more focussed on the hospital's reputation in a league table and performance management culture. This ends up often scapegoating the very professionals who are trying to work under sometimes impossible pressures. This leads to a culture of fear amongst staff and a lack of openness and learning to prevent future errors or shortcomings. These errors can also result in huge amounts of money being spent on negligence claims, estimated to be £13.6b in 2020/21 – that's 7% of the NHS budget. In fact, the litigation costs in the NHS are worse than in many states in the USA. I do believe that if we had a "learn not blame" culture, we would actually be able to create a safer system with less litigation, with more money available for patient care. We should emulate the aviation industry which saw a 75% reduction in safety incidents after adopting a no blame investigative culture.

Over 4 in 10 doctors report bullying and harassment at work, which also has an impact on the productivity of the workforce and patient care. Roger Kline has estimated that bullying is costing the NHS an estimated £2 billion a year from staff absence, stress and illness. The GMC Wellbeing report says burnout increases the risk of medical error by about 45–63%, which is significant.

The other problem we have in our health service, and to be frank, since its inception, is the organisational divide between primary and secondary care. This creates artificial and unnecessary barriers for patients who rightly expect their care to be in a coordinated whole system. And this inevitably results in fragmentation in care, duplication of effort, wastes resources and adversely affects patient care. For example, it makes no sense for a psychiatrist investigating a patient with memory loss to request a series of blood tests and an ECG but tell the patient to see their GP to do get these done – this should be able to be requested directly by the specialist preventing this duplication of work by the GP as well as preventing delays to treatment. Similarly, patients are routinely advised by specialists to see their GP for a prescription since the hospital prescribing budget does not cover the cost of the prescription, which is then borne by a separate GP budget. This waste GP time, but also delays care for the patient solely due to siloed prescribing budgets and incurs additional administrative costs to the NHS. It is estimated that 15 million GP appointments are wasted each year dealing with primary/secondary care interface administrative issues such as hospital generated tasks or appointment queries. These wasted appointments could instead be offered by GPs to patients who need medical care, and thereby improving access.

At the inception of the NHS, GPs were considered as "gatekeepers", referring patients to specialists. When I qualified as a GP 30 years ago, it was routine to refer patients with diabetes, chronic heart and respiratory conditions to hospital specialists, who would look after their ongoing care. Now, GPs manage such conditions often entirely in the community. The idea of a primary/secondary care divide is a misnomer, with GPs now very much co-providers of care together with their hospital colleagues. Similarly in the community, we have a separation between GP services and community nursing services, which means patients needing treatment at home are often caught in the crossfire of which services GPs provide and those of district nurses, resulting in fragmentation and delay.

The reality is that there are major fracture lines between the specialist, community and primary care teams and that is hugely inefficient and damaging. We have matured since 1948 and need to think and practise differently within a new modern collaborative paradigm.

I also believe that the other major issue for the NHS is that it is a system driven by politicians. Even within a single government electoral term, just changing the health secretary changes the policies of the health service. So when you consider the last three different health secretaries of the current government, each of them had quite different views. So you have a health service that's at the mercy of political whim. It is also at the mercy of electoral whim in terms of the political party that is elected. Every time you get a new government, it will come up with a new blueprint for the NHS, driven by electoral timescales and motives to appeal to public opinion rather than having an objective approach on how the health service should be run. One potential solution is setting up an independent Board (as is for the Bank of England) to set national policy based on objective health needs and without political interference or short term electoral timelines.

I: What's your view of the strengths of the NHS as a healthcare system?

CN: The most important strength the NHS has is that it provides free care at the point of access and is still based upon need not on the basis of a person's status or ability to pay. In fact, if a person had a road traffic accident or a heart attack, it would not matter whether the individual was a peer of the realm or a homeless person - the ambulance will take you to the hospital within the same priority status and you would end up being treated the same. So it is very much a fair system. Another important fact is that there's no financial transactions at the point of care which is different from many insurance-based systems or in other countries where you pay a co-payment fee,. Not having to pay generates trust between a patient and a doctor.

I'm reminded of when I sat my final medical school examinations, and a friend of mine persuaded me to sit the USA entrance examination (ECFMG) at the same time, saying there would be greater opportunities there. I passed and then in my first year as a junior doctor, I went for a holiday to the States for the first time to explore possibilities. I was just struck by how the whole system was based upon a business model when I met a few doctors. A family friend who was suffering from recurrent urinary infections asked me whether she should go back to see her doctor for an ultrasound scan. When I questioned why she asked me this, she said that she suspected he may requesting more investigations because he gets paid for each follow up. That was like an epiphany and I realised that I did not want to be a part of a system where patients doubt or question my motives as a doctor. That is the strength of the NHS - if I request a scan there is no financial gain to me and the decision is based only in the best interest of the patient within resource constraints and guidelines. This is fundamental to establishing mutual trust with patients.

Because the NHS is free at the point of access, it is also an exceptionally equitable system as has been repeatedly judged by the Commonwealth Fund. Patients do not default on their care due to cost constraints, and are not dissuaded from having treatment on the basis of cost, which is the phenomenon that is seen in many other nations, even those with state funded health services which charge a small fee or a co-payment for their care. In such systems, people on the lowest incomes or who are financially disadvantaged will inherently see accessing health as a cost barrier.

The other strength of the NHS is that it is a coordinated national service although I don't think it's coordinated enough. Institutes like NICE create policies and recommendations which set national standards. The public feel that they're being treated in a standardised manner. In many countries the system will actually be different in parts of the country because they're run by insurance companies and competing interests. There are also national specifications with regards to access to specialist and tertiary care, ensuring that every region in the UK is served by services such as cancer, renal and cardiac. As we saw during the pandemic, we can also have coordinated national responses to public health emergencies notwithstanding concerns about whether the government's response to Covid was right or wrong.

I: I agree that burnout is a major problem which then adds to pressure leading to more disengagement. Also inevitably maximum pressure from above falls on junior doctors who have the least power. You have mentioned changes in society, changes in professional roles, patient expectations and other factors so if you were redesigning the NHS today, how would you do it?

CN: One of the first things I would do is to free the NHS from policy making by politicians. I would design the NHS with people who are stakeholders: healthcare professionals who work within the NHS, who have relevant expertise, public health experts, people who understand healthcare systems, users of the service and others who can help create a health service based upon their experience. Ultimately the service is owned by the population as they pay for it. So the public should be aware of the realities of the constraints in delivery of healthcare in the face of increasing demands - this would create a much more appropriate level of understanding, as well as expectations. Yet the politicisation of the health service creates a lack of honesty and transparency with the public, with information tailored to suit media headlines and electoral success. A recent example is that in spite of clear calls for an independent workforce specification and strategy in the Health Bill of 2022, politicians chose to reject it. Why would you reject a strategy that tells you how many healthcare professionals you need in the health service? You wouldn't, for example, run Tesco by saying you don't know how many floor staff and cashiers you need. I believe that the government rejected this call because they knew that politically it would expose the extent of workforce shortages in the NHS, and identify a resource shortfall that they wouldn't want to be publicised.

I would create a truly independent Board or body which would specify the resources, workforce and infrastructure required to provide a comprehensive health service, to levels equivalent to other comparative EU nations. It would also provide independent scrutiny of the NHS and ensure the public were objectively informed. I realise that ultimately the government is accountable to the public for the provision of healthcare as a public service, but it will then have be honest about the resource, workforce and infrastructure requirements of the NHS and of any gaps and how it will address this.

As part of this honesty there should be a compact with the population about collective responsibility for fair and appropriate use of the common resource called the NHS where no one is left behind. If the public openly and explicitly knows from the top that we are desperately short of GPs – 2000 fewer today than in 2015 despite seeing tens of millions of more patients per year in this period- I believe they will understand these pressures, have realistic expectations and demand this workforce deficit is corrected. For example, the public did not blame the attendants in local petrol stations when we had a national petrol shortage. They knew that there was a shortage of lorry drivers.

We also must have a system that breaks down what has been up to now historic boundaries between primary, secondary, community and social care services. As I said earlier this is creating huge inefficiencies and adversely impacting on patient care with duplication and fragmentation. I see the current development of integrated care systems in England as partly a political sop. It's not really properly integrated. It's basically bringing people together around a table while the system inherently continues to be divided. A truly integrated system would not require patients to be having duplication of transactions for example between hospitals and general practices. You would not have mal-aligned incentives. You would not have Foundation Trusts having a board meeting purely about the performance and the financial position of that particular Trust in isolation. You would actually have systems of board meetings that looked at a sector-wide approach of how cross-sector resources can be used most effectively. I would actually break down those barriers and I would create service pathways of care where we bring together the various providers of care under one umbrella. And the aim would be to minimise duplication of effort and putting the patients' experience first. Once you start with that, you wouldn't transfer workload or cost from one sector to the other since it would all be part of a single overall budget. A coordinated single system reducing inefficiencies through synergistic collaborative arrangements which I believe would work really well.

As I previously stated, I would also create a new paradigm in NHS culture - a caring, supportive no blame culture that recognises the reality of pressures and constraints that staff work within, and that things will inevitably go wrong at times. A learning culture where staff feel free to speak out about their concerns or patient safety, in which the system welcomes and embraces these views as a means of ongoing quality improvement and reducing patient harm. Its aim would always be to identify how it can become better and safer rather than starting with whose fault it is.

This will make the NHS a safer place, as well as reducing costs of litigation for medical negligence. This would include learning from international models where there is no-fault compensation. I recently spoke to a doctor from the Netherlands, where serious untoward incidents are investigated in a way that doctors who may have been implicated are part of the investigation to help prevent a recurrence. This is because it's a proper no-blame, no-fault compensation approach. In the NHS healthcare workers who are implicated will feel dissuaded from speaking out due to fear of blame and litigation against them personally. Clearly there needs to be accountability where there is individual culpability or wilful neglect, but most errors in the NHS stem from systemic factors rather than solely from individuals.

We also require a radically different performance culture in the NHS, where politicians no longer create performance targets that result in perverse behaviour. It also requires a new type of NHS leadership, from health ministers cascaded down to NHS England, and leaders in NHS providers, who put the well-being of staff as their priority.

This investment in well-being will pay dividends, given the evidence that this will improve safety and productivity. This new NHS culture must eradicate experiences of bullying, racism and discrimination amongst the workforce, since not only is this wrecking the lives of so many healthcare staff, but it also is affecting workforce numbers and absenteeism. This will require leaders who are truly driven by values of inclusivity and equality and need to be appointed with these attributes.

In redesigning the NHS I would also make sure that prevention of ill health was really embedded at its heart with a strong public health infrastructure. There have been savage cuts to public health budgets in recent years, which is false economy, since by not preventing ill-health, it ends up costing the NHS more in treatment. This again is a victim of political running of the NHS and electoral timescales, since investment in public health results in change over longer periods than before the next general election. We must definitively address the wider determinants of health such as poverty, housing, unemployment. Again, we have silos of budgets covering these areas, separated from the NHS. For example, improving people's health would reduce those claiming disability benefits and reduce costs in the welfare sector. However, investment in the NHS will be seen as an additional cost pressure, even though it may actually end up reducing the cost to the taxpayer overall by lowering benefit claims.

I: I agree about silos and have talked about it before but it is a major task, so how do we bring it together? How would you see that working?

CN: Firstly, there needs to be a genuine change in culture and mindset of those in power – starting at government- recognising how damaging and counter-productive the current silos in the NHS are. In fact, for the government, it is both costing the NHS more with wasted expense in fragmentation and duplication, but also adversely impacting on patient care.

There then needs to be proper structural changes in terms of the way in which the NHS operates and ending its disparate competing funding streams – so that we break down the boundaries between different sectors, with proper coordinated and collaborative care for patients. For example the current ICSs could be redefined to commission and fund services within a single pathway in which the hospital specialist, the GP, community services and social care would operate as single coordinated service. Pathway commissioned services would direct patients to the most relevant healthcare professional rather than the current ping-pong between GP and hospital specialist and would be driven to improve the patient experience without duplication. So a specialist requesting investigations before the next follow-up outpatient appointment would directly request this in the community, rather than asking the GP to do so, and also able to prescribe using electronic links with local community pharmacists. Because the budget would be integrated, this would have no cost implications on the hospital as compared to it being done by the GP. So patients will not be bouncing between providers. In Tower Hamlets, there is an integrated renal service for chronic kidney disease (CKD) where the GP and hospital doctor have a shared patient record system. In that setting the specialist looks at the record, adds to it with management decisions as a shared approach with GPs- rather than the traditional approach of a GP referral, outpatient clinic appointment, and then a recommendation back to the GP of what to do next. This has apparently stopped outpatient flows by 90% because patients are being managed as one team. Also the whole relationship becomes teamwork and there's no game playing or blame.

Indeed, I feel as healthcare professionals life could be so much more rewarding when we all feel we are "on the same side", and in some ways resurrects our beginnings as medical students when we were all part of one cohort, before we branched out to our specialties after qualifying as doctors. It would be so motivating to be part of a system where I as a GP felt genuinely part of a team that included community nurses and hospital specialists, with all of us playing to each other strengths, and the system supporting us to work together without duplication of effort, and supported by technology that made our relationships seamless.

I: You talked about the next 50–75 years of the NHS, do you think it has a future?

CN: I definitely believe and hope it has a future but only if there is a will to stock take where we are and address current issues and be bold and redefine the way it operates in keeping with its founding principles. As the father of the NHS Aneurin Bevan said: "The NHS will last as long as there are folk left with faith to fight for it".

I do believe that the founding principles are as relevant today as they were in 1948. I do not accept the arguments that these principles no longer apply or that the NHS is unaffordable or that we need to think of patient charges for services. The NHS is a highly efficient healthcare system, with administrative costs far lower than comparative nations who operate for example insurance based systems. It is equitable by nature, based on need not ability to pay.

The glaring impediment afflicting the NHS is lack of resources- both in terms of workforce numbers and physical infrastructure such as beds grossly below equivalent nations such as France and Germany. Many point to our European neighbours as having better health outcomes, using this as an argument for the NHS no longer being fit for purpose. However, if those European countries were to be stripped of tens of thousands of doctors, hospital beds, and force GPs to consult at short 10 minute appointments, their outcomes would also worsen.

Indeed, changing the NHS into one based on an insurance model would simply exacerbate its problems, with more spent on administrative transaction costs and even less money available for direct patient care.

The NHS is also affected by wider political and fiscal policy, which results in health inequalities, poverty, unemployment all of which add pressure on the NHS. These wider determinants of health must also be addressed for the future sustainability of the NHS.

I: You have touched upon workforce issues and related difficulties and specialisation; do you think there is any mileage in doing some kind of combined training across disciplines so people are aware of what their respective roles are? Often medical school training is in a silo but as soon as that training has finished, one is expected to work in a team and sometimes even lead it which means changing your mindset completely and working through that.

CN: Absolutely. When I trained the model of care was largely medical. There was no such thing as a nurse being able to even prescribe. The truth is that we are working in a very different environment now with other healthcare professionals doing work that doctors previously used to provide. Nurses can do biopsies, endoscopies and can autonomously manage minor conditions in accident and emergency units. In general practice, we have a growing multi-professional skill mix, with advance care practitioners, pharmacists, physiotherapists, paramedics and physicians associates seeing patients as part of a general practice team. This is vital to support GP workload, but even with this assistance, we are desperately short of doctors in the NHS. Therefore I don't see the multi-professional workforce threatening the role and value of doctors, but complementing us to be able to use our time purposefully working at the top of our licence doing the things that only doctors can do.

We should therefore reorganise training in a multi-professional and multi-skilled environment in a way that did not exist in 1948. I do not believe that this new model requires fewer doctors – in fact we need many more- but it is about changing the role of doctors. Demands on healthcare are increasing exponentially around the world. We are going to have to work by necessity in teams where other professionals can competently do many of the things that doctors used to do previously but did not need to be done by a doctor. The long and comprehensive medical training that we undergo results in medical professionals who have a unique set of skills which should be used at the highest possible levels and not at their lowest level. I don't want to go back to the days where as a GP I was spending an hour a day signing repeat prescriptions - -this is now all done by our practice pharmacists who also manage chronic conditions such as diabetes and asthma competently. I do not share the fear that some people have that this is about replacing skilled doctors with cheaper labour. On the contrary I think that the role of the doctor would flourish more by being able to have more time to do what only doctors can and should do.

I: The pandemic has taught us that it is perfectly possible to do certain things through online consultations and use of technology and for patients to also manage their own care.

CN: I believe that there has to be a very mature discussion on how to best use technology to its fullest extent in a way that will benefit both patients and healthcare professionals. There have been huge advances in IT over the decades, even in my time as a doctor. I qualified as a GP over 30 years ago, when we only had paper records – we are now fully computerised and fully paperless, with our GP IT providing us with clinical prompts and clinical decision support, and safety alerts when we prescribe. Patients themselves now self monitor their blood pressure. AI is coming-of-age, with evidence that it can at times be even more accurate in reading some radiological scans than the human eye. Some operations are now being safely done by robotic surgery. I can now as a GP issue a prescription electronically and instantly send it to any pharmacy in England near the patient, even when they are on holiday.

We must try and build on these technological advancements in an equitable way. We do not want digital exclusion and must make sure that there is provision of training, equipment and access to all who are able and willing to use digital technology, but also where they cannot, that traditional methods of care and support continue, so that no one is disadvantaged.

Technology is not only for those who are technically savvy or young and mobile. Assistive technology and machine learning such as Alexa-enabled voice commands can help bed-bound patients to be lifted on a hoist, etc. rather than having a carer come in. We know that robots can reduce loneliness in people at home performing simple tasks, playing music, etc. These things are already happening and are actually working.

Digital technology such as consultations on mobile phones can also improve equitable access, such as people who may not be able to leave home for a number of reasons including caring responsibilities, those working in jobs where they are unable to take time off work or are travelling, such as lorry drivers. It is not an either/or solution but use of technology can facilitate greater access to care for some.

AI is also now a reality, and it is vital that research and developments occur to ensure equity from gender to race. Neither does this need to threaten doctors – especially given the level workforce shortages and the increasing demands on medical care. For example there was concern that AI will make radiologists redundant. When I met representatives of The Royal College of Radiologists they acknowledged the role of AI and in fact felt it would free them to do more interventional work bringing them more in touch with patients. It's about adapting and changing our roles with technological advancements so that we can be enabled as doctors to work at the top of our game in a modern paradigm.

The pandemic also highlighted the huge potential for patients managing their own care. Although we have had a pulse oximeters is for decades, it took the pandemic to demonstrate its value in patients with respiratory symptoms routinely measuring their own oxygen levels at home .There is immense scope for patients to self manage minor ailments, reducing unnecessary demand on doctors. The pandemic accelerated home blood pressure monitoring with patients sending their readings to their GP surgery for advice and management - prior to that patients routinely took time out of their lives, and visited their GP simply to have their blood pressure checked. Patients can also effectively self manage chronic conditions, if assisted with easily understandable and guided information. The use of the NHS app, could be optimised. For example, patients with diabetes who are making frequent appointments to see me for their results could access these results directly from their smartphones with automated information on interpreting the result and also advice on management.

Patients who want to speak to their GP or clinician must always still be able to do so, and those unwilling or unable to use new technology must continue to have traditional access so that there is equity- indeed patients using technology in this way would actually free up staff time for other patients.

This is ultimately about patient empowerment in improving their own health and outcomes.

I: I agree with you that things are changing. The pandemic has taught us that we can do things differently and patients would accept that. Thanks Chaand, is there anything else that we have not covered or you would like to add?

CN: I think I've covered it. Thanks very much.

Note

1 https://www.bma.org.uk/advice-and-support/nhs-delivery-and-workforce/the-future/caring-supportive-collaborative-a-future-vision-for-the-nhs

10 Baroness Julia Neuberger

Baroness Julia Neuberger is an Emerita Rabbi. She was chair of King's Fund and is now a crossbench peer. She has been heavily involved in healthcare policy and management throughout her career. In the 1990s, she was chair of the Camden and Islington Community Trust and she has been closely involved with national reports on the Liverpool Care Pathway and the Mental Health Act Review. She has written widely. She is currently the chair of UCL NHS Foundation Trust.

Interview

I: Thanks very much for agreeing to be interviewed. You're currently chair of the UCL Foundation Trust. That puts you in a great position for this interview both from your current role and pastoral role as well as Past Chair of King's Fund. The idea is to look at where we are with the NHS coming up to its 75th anniversary and where we go in the next 25 years or so. Of course no one can predict the future but the aim is to look at the current state and check out the strengths and weaknesses of the NHS. You have seen the questions and we are not going through each question as is but a general discussion about your views and observations. One of the things that really worries me at the moment is that the NHS does not seem to be working efficiently.

JN: Well, it depends upon what you mean by efficiently. It works incredibly efficiently when you look at how, for instance, emergency departments work. They work incredibly hard and incredibly efficiently. The problems arise, for example, if you can't unload an ambulance into an emergency department, the emergency department then gets swallowed up by that. If you can't unload the ambulance because there isn't the capacity, because when they want to move people from the emergency department into a bed, say, an acute medical unit, there aren't any beds. And the reason there aren't any beds is that the acute medical unit can't send them to another ward

DOI: 10.4324/9781003382188-10

because the wards are all, at least in part, full of people who are ready to go home or at least ready to go into some form of either home or residential care, but need huge social care support which may not be readily available. And we haven't solved social care. So if I really wanted to do something about the efficiency of the NHS, I would solve social care.

I: That was going to be one of my questions in terms of integration of health and social care. But also, one of the big challenges has been the relationship between mental health and physical health, and they seem to be into two separate orbits.

JN: We always think of everything in silos. We always do it partly because that is the way human beings are. So the whole idea of having integrated care systems was to try and bring services closer together. We all supported that because this is the right thing to do. So mental health to physical health, social care, to healthcare, etc. all need to come together. At the moment though it is not turning out like that. My own view is that integrating, not necessarily integrating the services, but integrating how you commission and integrating how you think about them is the key. We are not anywhere near that. If I were Secretary of State for Health or maybe if I were Prime Minister, I would be looking at social care. And that would be a combination of public funding and people having to fund it by themselves, and that will free up some of the hospital capacity. Then let's look at mental health and the extent to which people who have long-term mental health issues get very poor physical health care. Let's think about why that is and look at the silos and then think about the way to solve that. If we solve social care for people who have long-term mental health issues that can really support people to live in the community and access decent physical care? So can we stop categorising and labelling in that way and looking at what the individual's needs are as opposed to being labelled as a mental health patient? But I think you need to solve social care before you even can do that.

I: Thanks, that is spot-on. There are other things such as sometimes rigid borders between primary and secondary care and the other one is public health, which sits in a separate silo. Covid pandemic has taught us that we need to bring all these together somehow.

JN: We agreed that we would do this through the integrated care system. The question is, are they going to be serious about the health of their populations? Or are the integrated care boards going to be just managing the performance of the NHS? The integrated care system is supposed to be looking at the population health needs of the population concerned. I actually think that's really important. We ought to be doing that. I should be very, very, very pleased if we managed to do it. On the boundary between primary and secondary care, we have a primary health care crisis in that we're losing GPs at a massive rate. People don't want to go into being a GP. I think we're going to have to rethink the model because at the moment at least part of the pressure, not all of it by any means, in emergency departments is people not getting GP appointments or not wanting to get a GP appointment because of the wait. A lot of emergency departments are being used for primary care and that's absurd. We ought to be able to solve at least a part of that by investing in primary care, using nurses more, physician associates more, and probably somewhat changing the model.

I: That is related to the way we deliver services. And again, Covid pandemic has illustrated that you can use telehealth and e-health much more efficiently. On occasion when I have contacted the GP surgery through e-contact, they have come back within 2 hours and things have been done, investigations or prescriptions, within 24 hours. So somehow that kind of mixed care approach works.

JN: You may be getting better service than some of us ....

I: I must say that I did have lots of concerns about telehealth, particularly in terms of confidentiality and privacy. When you ring somebody, you don't know who else is in the room listening. How do we balance the demands on the NHS? It is a clear tension between demands and responsibility so how do we manage that? Demand is rising, whereas the funds are not enough.

JN: Well, there will never be enough money to do everything you want to do. And think about what we spend on diagnostics compared with, say, even 20 years ago. Everybody having MRIs or scans or whatever they did. So we have bumped up the costs because we can do more and in cancers, for instance, we can do a huge amount more, but it's very expensive. So health professionals may want to say that patients should take more responsibility for their own health. Well, you can say that till you are blue in the face, but it's not going to happen. So actually you have to think about it the other way. What we have to do is say that these are the things that you will get via the NHS and we'll have to make it easier to get things quickly. So walk-in diagnostics are a really good idea. Some sort of walk-in primary care is going to be really important, they may be seen by a nurse rather than a doctor. But that's fine. Then you can be seen by the one doctor on-site if needed. You can't just say to people, we have a National Health Service, but you can't use it because that's just not tolerable. And health professionals get very irritated by people coming to the emergency departments with the most ridiculous things, for example, ingrown toenail. But the truth of the matter is that you can make it more difficult and you can send them to see the nurse or whatever. But that's what patients are going to do. They don't know how else to access anything. We've never succeeded in getting the public to use pharmacists more. But we should have done it.

I: That is a very good point because pharmacists do get five years training.

JN: They are incredibly knowledgeable.

I: Yes. That is the other challenge. How do we use other professions such as nurses, pharmacists and physician associates? You have touched upon their roles. What are your views about specialists and generalists?

JN: You have to have a generalist, don't you? So that people can go see someone and explain and the generalist can either deal with it themselves or refer them on to the right specialist. So you have to have generalists and they do not necessarily always need to be doctors. So you have to think about this differently.

I: One of the big challenges, particularly in medicine, is that it comes down to the status thing. Also as some colleagues have mentioned, it is about tribalism. Every body wants to be a specialist partly because of money and reimbursements. Specialists will say that I am a right knee specialist and not a left knee one.

JN: Yes. You are going to have more and more of that because in fact, with more precision surgery, you're actually only going to be able to deal with the left knee rather than the right knee or whatever. I don't think you can do much about that. I think the trend is still more specialisation. I don't think we want to go to the American model where while you are at home and say, I've got a stomach ache and I need to see a gastroenterologist. I still think you're better off seeing a generalist, a general physician of some sort or other. But the general physician doesn't necessarily need to be a doctor.

I: Going back to what you were saying about the redesign of the NHS, and let's assume it didn't exist and you were going to set something up. What would you do?

JN: I don't think I could answer that question because it has existed for nearly 75 years. In a funny British way it is a religion. What does everybody believe in? And they believe in the NHS. They are very critical of it but they believe in it. I remember Rudolph Klein writing this article about the NHS whether it was a church or a garage. It is more like a church than a garage. I don't have an answer. What would you do? You would still have to set up some kind of healthcare system which would be paid for by some insurance system if it wasn't paid for by the public purse. It makes no difference. Other countries have got similar problems.

I: As you mentioned part of the challenge really is the integration between various components of the NHS and social care but how do we pay for that? And if it is truly integrated then it makes sense and far easier to move people according to their needs.

JN: But unless you're going to put a huge amount of public money into the NHS and social care, that isn't going to happen. Even if you have much better relationships between health services and social care services, unless the money is really huge which is highly unlikely. There will always have to be some form of personal contribution to social care. So you don't completely solve it. If you wanted a totally national health and social care service then maybe it is possible. But I don't see that coming. I don't see anybody being willing to pay for very, very expensive care.

I: One of the things that struck me in the NHS is that it is not very good at workforce planning and it lurches from crisis to crisis.

JN: It is not the NHS really is it? It is the government.

I: It is interesting that when the Secretary of State pops up to say that by so-and-so date we will have 5000 extra GPs.

JN: It is rubbish and everybody knows it is rubbish. Actually Jeremy Hunt, as Chair of the Health Select Committee, reported yesterday that workforce planning is the biggest issue in the NHS and in primary care workforce funding is one of the major issues. Did you see that from yesterday?

I: No, I haven't seen that.

JN: Have a look at that. That's the Health Select Committee report. Have a look at that because it says exactly that.

I: One of the things that really intrigues me is the number of doctors who are dropping out as soon as they finish their foundation year training. It used to be about 3–4%, and I think it's now about 11%. They're either taking time out or they're going abroad, but there are also other related issues that I don't think anybody has dared tackle that younger generation want a much better work-life balance, and 60% of medical students are women. Their priorities are likely to be different. So you basically need one and a half people to fill one post.

JN: I don't think the old system where people worked ridiculous hours was very good for patients. The dropout rate is a different thing. People get much of their training paid for, even though people do pay part of the cost. They don't pay the full cost or anything like the full cost of actual training. So if people don't stay or do stay five years or eight years in the system, one would say that they have to be charged more because they have taken the training and not used it.

I: I trained in Armed Forces Medical College in Poona. Half of my class had to sign a bond to go into the services. The rest of us had to pay our own way. Some could join a short service commission, whereas others did so for their whole career.

JN: I think it is unreasonable to say you are going to do it for life, but I do think you can say, but you must do it for a minimum period of time.

I: I have often urged politicians to be frank with the public with a pie chart to say that for every pound that is spent in the NHS, the distribution of costs towards staffing, investigations, beds, etc. are really clear. There seems to be a degree of reluctance.

JN: That's easy enough to see from the accounts of any NHS organisation. The NHS is made up of its parts, so I don't think there's a difficulty finding out where the money goes. I don't think that's difficult.

I: What do you see as the future of the NHS?

JN: Well I think we will have an NHS. I think the public loves it and I think politically you couldn't get rid of it. I think that it depends on what kind of government we have. There are likely various attempts to get us to pay a bit more for it. There may even be attempts to get us to pay at the point of use. We do know that if you get people to pay at the point of use, then the most deprived won't use it. And that's a real problem, particularly if you're taking a public health approach. I think it will exist in some form for the next 25 years. Whether it will be exactly as it is now, I don't know. There will be a lot more telehealth, a lot more telephone conversations and a lot more online consultations. I think the idea of you going into a GP surgery will almost go. I think that that model will go and I suspect the outpatient, as we know it, will largely go.

I: People will need to see a clinician if they needed a physical examination or a blood test.

JN: Yes. Then you will go to a specialist centre to get your physical examination, a blood test. You will go to a community diagnostic centre where you can have a blood test or you can have your CAT scan.

I: That's a good point.

JN: And that's coming.

I: Certainly as the pandemic has hit, the NHS has struggled to cope and waiting lists have burgeoned and there was a piece in the paper yesterday or day before about the number of people who've gone private to have their surgeries done. Do you think that there's a danger that we would reach a tipping point where the government might say to people that you can afford to pay so go private?

JN: No. I don't think the government will say you can afford to pay so you go and have it privately because they can't afford to do that. If they carry on saying the NHS is a universal service, I think it may get to the point where it's much more likely that those who can afford it will go and have their elective surgery privately. And I don't think that's so terrible, provided you have a reasonable service for those who can't afford it.

I: There is an implicit social contract between patient and medicine and medicine and government and patients and government tripartite contract so how do we ensure that people are aware of it?

JN: We don't. We don't make the contract explicit. But people know that if they need care, they can get it. And how easily can they get this and how soon can they get it? If it's something that isn't elective, it's pretty good. The cancer waiting times at the moment are really worrying post-Covid, but that will, I think, sort itself out to some extent. The assumption that if you really need care, you can get it will remain. The question what will happen about some of the elective stuff will remain. I think that assumption will remain. You can't write a contract.

I: No.

JN: When I was at King's Fund, we tried to set out values for the NHS for the 50th anniversary. Actually it is quite important that the NHS states what it is about, what its values are and what it is for. I still think it's quite important for the NHS to have a defined and clear value set. The idea of a contract with the public I don't think will work, but I do think that people need to know what they're entitled to.

I: Social contract is not explicit but it is an implicit one. Medicine has become much more complex and technical.

JN: And physical examination happens much less. I can't think when I last had somebody actually physically examined me, it doesn't happen.

I: Through the BMA, we did a survey of mental health and wellbeing of doctors and medical students, and the burnout rates in medical students were horrendous. When we interviewed them, they came up with various explanations, and top of the list was that medicine is too technical and they felt that they did not come in to become technicians.

JN: Well, actually, medical students did come in to be technicians. They would know because that has been the case for some time. Even nursing has become very much more technical. People don't recognise that because a lot of the things that nurses used to do are being done by healthcare assistants these days. Our senior nurses are giving chemotherapy. In some situations they're doing biopsies and gastroscopies. Increasingly, it is likely that gastroscopies will be replaced by pill cameras so it is a change. Practice of medicine changes all the time. Medical students may not like being technicians, but that is the direction of travel in medicine. I'm quite worried about the wellbeing of doctors because I do think doctors suffered very, very badly during Covid. They had a really terrible time. I think the ones who had the best time were the ones who were deeply involved and were at the cutting edge. For a lot of people, it was very hard to function and now they are left with these huge waiting lists trying to manage these. So I think that's difficult.

I: Do you think that perhaps as senior professionals, we are not conveying the current state of medicine about what has changed?

JN: But it's very obvious what has changed? It is very obvious. You go to the emergency department and you will get a lot of stuff that's quite technical very quickly.

I: In terms of training, although we are all expected to work in teams, our training is quite often very separate. Do you have a view as to how we can change that?

JN: Not really, because you have to do the various bits. I do think that an awful lot of medical students are much happier about the quality of the teaching they're getting now that you hear a lot about that. And we have a lot of students. I particularly meet with students at Whittington, and they're really having a nice time. I think they're really enjoying it. You have to do different subjects. I would like to see medical students having to do more of some specific subjects, particularly. For example, we are not very good at pain management and students don't know enough about how to deal with pain. They don't know about that. And I think we should. There are some overarching things. I think it would be good to be able to do more of. And I quite like some of the American models. I like the patient-doctor model they've got at Harvard Medical School where, you know, you spend quite a lot of time as a medical student, actually, with patients living with patients, sometimes with long-term conditions. I think there is quite a lot to be said for that approach. I think people need more often more practical experience.

I: One of the things that I would like to see is teaching psychiatry from day 1 of medical school rather than in year 4.

JN: Absolutely. I think for a lot of things you need to have a mental health overview. You need to have some understanding about social factors such as what debt and deprivation do to mental health and wellbeing, what I call social medicine. So a social medicine overview needs to be there right from the beginning.

I: During my medical school training in India, we were taught preventive and social medicine and as part of the internship we had to do three months, but most of it was focussed on infection control, vaccinations, nutrition, etc. but nothing on mental health.

JN: I think people need to have that as an overview right the way through that. That's a really interesting idea.

I: I think then you can link social determinants and geopolitical determinants and teaching people how to educate. You have touched upon some of the interesting innovations such as community diagnostic clinics and health centres. Are there any examples of good clinical practice that you think we need to teach medical students?

JN: The thinking behind palliative care is transformational. But I'd like to see some of that thinking going away from end of life into generalised thinking about medicine. That's one example. I have seen some absolutely amazing work on cancer centres where you have some complementary therapy available as well as the absolutely intense chemotherapies and radiotherapies, surgery, etc. I love the way that the cancer centre works here at UCL where you get lots of other things as well as traditional cancer therapies. I think there are loads of fantastic individual practices. I think the use of arts in and music helps change that perspective and enables us to tolerate pain much better. I just think we're really quite bad at using what we've learned from specific things and generalising them.

I: Is there anything else that you think that we haven't covered? Anything further you'd like to add?

JN: I think that I've probably covered more or less what I want to say. There is a real issue about the politicisation of the NHS. I have to say that on the record because I think it's very difficult if every Secretary of State thinks that they've got to make some changes. So they rearrange the deck chairs and make it extremely difficult to run a system. People in charge politically want to show that they are doing something when it's very difficult for them to know what to do. That really is a problem for the NHS. And I'd rather that the politicians concentrate on things like workforce planning than rearranging the deck chairs. That is really, really important.

I: Thanks very much for your time, that is incredibly helpful.

11 Dr Max Pemberton

Max Pemberton is a doctor, working full time in the National Health Service (NHS) in mental health. He is also a journalist and a columnist for the Daily Mail, writing weekly on politics, cultural and social issues, ethics, mental health and the NHS. Prior to moving to the Mail, he was a columnist for the Daily Telegraph for 12 years. He writes a monthly short story for Readers Digest as well as a column for them and is a regular contributor to the Spectator. He has written five books. His first, Trust Me I'm a Junior Doctor, was serialised as Radio 4 Book of the Week. His latest book is a children's book called *The Marvellous Adventure of Being Human*.

Interview

I: The aim of the interview is really to focus on the NHS. You are both a journalist and a clinician in the NHS. So if we start with your view of the state of play in the NHS at this time?

MP: Well, I think it's difficult to give a really comprehensive overview at the moment, because we are still seeing the aftershocks of Covid– both the virus, and also our response to the virus in terms of things like lockdown. I think the NHS was in a fairly perilous state before the lockdown and before the pandemic. And now I think it is in quite dire straits really, for a number of reasons, not least the fact that it was just about managing to sort of limp along and keep its head above water. And it was really that we were sort of living hand-to-mouth with that. And of course, now we have essentially pressed pause on the NHS with loss of routine services for nearly two years. We were just about coping and now we have a huge backlog. Interestingly we talk about the NHS as though it's some sort of a single blob. But of course there are variations. Within the NHS there are some things that tend to work very well and are very well resourced and then there are other things and other areas which are not well resourced and which do not work well. And so

DOI: 10.4324/9781003382188-11

I think it makes it difficult to give a general overview of it. I think one of the things that tend to happen is the people who are very passionately pro-NHS will look at things that it does very well and areas that are really successful. As it happens these areas are likely to be very well resourced and use that as evidence. And then on the other hand are people who are more critical of the NHS perhaps from a political, ideological point of view, who are more opposed to a national health service, and who will then look at areas that are really failing and then use that for attacking the service. Because the NHS is such an enormous organisation and covers so much areas of our lives, whatever you want to argue, you can always find evidence of it.

I: What do you see as its strengths and weaknesses?

MP: Well, I think that if you are in extremis, it is fantastic. I think that if you have a complex case which requires lots of expert input, it is fantastic. And its structure is unlike the private sector, where people often have a vested interest and tendency to over- investigate. And I have seen lots of people who have slightly obscure things wrong with them or unusual constellations of symptoms who then go up and down Harley Street seeing specialist after specialist and waste a year or longer having every kind of extraordinary test. They may not have anyone who is going to step back and take an overview putting all these ideas together to actually what's going on. One of the amazing thing in the NHS is having an MDT (multi-disciplinary team) working approach in severe illnesses such as cancer and these areas tend to do quite well. There may be a very small number of treatments in the private sector that you cannot get in the NHS but apart from that, you are going to get pretty good world-class health-care if you are very unwell. Then, things like intensive care you will not get that privately. Even things like accident and emergency are very rarely available in private facilities, perhaps urgent care for cuts and bumps, etc. only in some private settings. If you are in a road traffic accident, it's the NHS that is going to be there for you. That is an enormous strength because when people are incredibly unwell, they want someone to be there and hold their hand and give them good care. Unfortunately it (NHS) very much falls down in several areas. I think it's in the minor things like hernia, cataract, joint replacement which are often seen in older people and also less prioritised within the health service. And yet we know that often these so-called minor things will have really detrimental impact in the long term on people's health and also their mental wellbeing. If you are an older person, at home with relatively poor mobility and you cannot read newspaper or watch television because of cataracts, that is going to have a profound impact on your mental health. We tend to compartmentalise these things. So cataracts are a minor operation. It is not seen as a priority. We need to protect people who are going blind and focus on some catastrophic eye injury and so on and we are going to put money there and we are not going to think about a cataract. And so, I think over time, these kinds of relatively minor operations are cut back and ignored. The fact that though they might be relatively minor procedures, they have a massive impact on people's lives and functioning. And we see that within who is going privately. If you are a general surgeon and you do hernia, hips, knee, varicose veins, etc. you would have seen your private practice bloom. I think it is a tragedy because it is a basic misunderstanding of healthcare. We know that minor things can still have a big impact on people's mental health and wellbeing. It also undermines fundamentally the NHS in the kind of model of care. I worry that it is a slippery slope that once you start saying that a hip or a hernia operation is not that important, where do you start drawing the line about what is important and what is not and then what should be a priority. I think minor procedures and minor ailments tend to fall down. Also at the moment, Accident & Emergency (A&E) are under enormous pressures. I think the basic model of A & E is actually very good. I am afraid to say that at present general practice is fundamentally letting patients down for a number of very complex reasons. It is not as simple as just saying we need more money, we pay doctors more or even we just need more doctors. I think that what we're seeing now is actually a very complex set of circumstances. For example, we are actually recruiting 50–70% women into medical schools. And that is great. It is good to have equitable split. But what people haven't realised that any workforce planning needs to take that into account so that people can take time out to bring up families and how gender roles tend to be acted out. Women may wish to work or return to work part-time and are likely to be attracted towards General Practice for flexibility. In view of individuals choosing to work part-time, we should have been recruiting twice as many doctors to account for that. Regrettably we have not been doing that. So we are now seeing a legacy of mismanagement of the medical workforce. It may be that is a difficult conversation to have. When I have written about or talked about the feminisation of medicine, people get a bit twitchy about it and accuse me of being sexist. I am not saying that women should not be doctors; what I am saying is that the evidence shows that they tend to not work full time and therefore we need to account for that. Or we need to create structures as teachers have that the working hours are such that they can provide child and family care if required. We may need to be similar to as anaesthetists have done, where people finish work at three so that they can pick up their kids from school. Similarly we may look at restructuring general practice in order to accommodate people taking care of families perhaps working in shifts. From readers, family members and my own contact general practice remains a matter of concern for people. They feel very let down by GPs and there is a lot of anger and hostility towards general practice in a way that there is not towards (other) doctors in general, and I think it's wrong to dismiss that. It is general practice, and not necessarily individual GP for that.

I: I think you're absolutely right. It is really surprising that the work force planning in this country has been abysmal. Changing the tack slightly, if you were setting up the NHS today, how would you do it?

MP: Well, my answer to that question has changed quite dramatically over the last few years. There were several things I would do. I have become slightly more disillusioned with the overall model as it currently works – or if it doesn't work sometimes – and also the way that clinicians operate within that and also the way patients use it. I think from a patient use perspective, people have – and it's totally understandable – become complacent. I think they like the idea of the NHS. They are very grateful when it helps them, but fundamentally they don't appreciate quite how much things cost, its complexity and how their choices have knock-on effects. For example, I went to see somebody who'd been referred by GP last week and I turned up and this is a two-hour assessment and she wasn't there and they were very apologetic. But I had spent an hour beforehand talking to the GP. I had spent some time reading all the notes and so on. Also, it took me 40 minutes to get there and 40 minutes to get back. So it was a four-hour appointment but actually ended up taking me nearly the whole day as I had blocked out periods afterwards to do my paperwork, which I couldn't do. I feel very hesitant saying this because it is fundamentally against the founding principle of the NHS whether a financial element needs to be introduced, not to make people pay directly for the actual services they receive because they have already done that. Whether it is worth thinking about introducing a penalty for missing appointments as that affects other patients too. When the NHS was first started people had in living memory of what it was like to have to pay for doctors to be called out, what it was like to have to pay for medication and so on. And the choices you had to make. My great grandmother had to call her GP because she developed a tooth abscess. If you needed to have your tooth removed, you were charged for the call out. But then they would call for the anesthetist so she didn't have anesthetic because she did not have the money for it. So she had a tooth extraction without an anesthetic. So when the NHS is introduced and everything is free, people are likely to be overwhelmed by that; it was an amazing thing. We have just forgotten that – it is no longer part of our collective consciousness at all. And so as a resource, I think it has slipped away from people's consciousness how quite valuable it is and what a privilege it is. I think therefore, introducing an element of financial penalties to disincentivise people from just not turning up is the only way to address the complacency that has crept into the NHS from the user point of view. So I wonder, if there is an opportunity to look at that if you fail to attend an appointment you'll be fined £20. If you turn up to A & E and for non-medical or non-urgent problem you will be fined £10 or £15 – a nominal fee to cover the cost of actually processing something that essentially was either wasted or was actually not necessary. I would also very much be up for charging people who end up drunk in A & E. That is just a particular bugbear of mine, having spent many years working in A & E. I love a drink myself but I have never got to the stage where I am so drunk that I need A & E. Often these are not the people who got drunk and fallen over or had an accident. These are people that are just so drunk they need to be taken to hospital. To me, that is extraordinary level of drinking. I think that things like this tend to overwhelm NHS resources. It is only a very small area but it goes to show that people need to take more responsibility for their actions. I think one of the things that's difficult is that kind of contract that society has with the NHS, and equally the NHS has with society. We have abused it or it has become muddied and a contract like that only works if everyone is taking responsibility for their health. Otherwise if everyone thinks that somebody else is going to sort it all out, we will end up paying for that person and then it disincentivises anyone else for ever taking responsibility for their health. So I wonder if there is an element of punishment we can introduce. I use that word quite cautiously, but punishing negative behaviours that we would rather discourage, but equally importantly nudging people towards making more positive choices. And so I wonder within the NHS if there is a wider thing that we could do about people who are exercising more, eating healthily and so on and so on, thereby encouraging them. At the moment, it's not really encouraged.

Also on a general point, I would merge immediately mental health trust and physical health trusts. The first thing I would do. I think that all that does is perpetuate the idea of there being a division between mental health and physical health. I find it hugely odd that we have this kind of parity of esteem that people talk about and yet we have quite literally enshrined within the health service this difference. It seems really odd. We know that mental illness is hugely costly to treat. And the current model that we have, which is this kind of mixed economy of care that was introduced in the last 20 years and where hospitals are encouraged and supposedly financially independent means that the mental health trusts are starting off at a disadvantage because the nature of the population itself that they are serving starts at a massive disadvantage. If you provide cancer care, you can specialise, and you can outsource services, you can make money. So there are ways of monetising the service, but it is very hard to do that in mental health.

I think it is massively unfair for mental health so that is the first thing I will do. I also feel that the current way that the health service manages GPs isn't particularly helpful. If I were starting all over again, if I was Bevan, I would have been very careful with GPs. I feel that it has not been very helpful having GPs as essentially separate franchises. It has been very, very difficult. There are GP partners who are so desperate they have just handed the keys back to the CCG (Clinical Commissioning Groups) because they want to go part-time or go salaried.

I think that that we should bring primary care into the NHS properly and integrate it into the service fully. I am also quite worried about dentistry. We have to look carefully at what has happened there. I think it's really quite catastrophic. And if we talk to any dentists and they have loads of brilliant ideas on what to do and none of it is to maintain the current system, I think we should include dentistry within the healthcare service properly, as opposed to it being this kind of strange annexe.

I: Right. You have touched upon it already but can you say a bit more about patients' rights versus responsibilities?

MP: Well. Essentially the NHS is a nationalised risk pooling approach, which is very similar to any insurance model works. So if I join health insurers, they decide what level of risk I am. I enter that pool of people that everyone is paying in and based on how risky I am to need to take out from that pot of money that we all pay in. That is what decides the level of contribution I make. The thing that's difficult about a nationalised model is that one cannot do that with every single person. It's too complicated. So essentially we all have to pay basically a flat fee or taxation relative to our income. So the difficulty is that whereas within a private healthcare insurance model, there is an incentive for example to not smoke, not be overweight, to exercise, etc. because that behaviour change is reflected in what I pay in, how much I have to pay. We don't have that.

So I see the difficulties. Therefore we have to make it very explicit to people that even though they are paying the same as everyone else, actually the choices they make are putting them at an increased risk and that also means that they would disproportionately take out of the pot. At the moment, we have to be very wary and scared of saying that, as it comes across as nanny state-ish, pejorative and quite unpleasant, but actually it is fundamental to the NHS. Obesity will cripple the NHS long before any politician does. They will keep on pumping money and the NHS will limp along but it will be people who can't stop eating cake are likely to kill the NHS. And yet very few clinicians are prepared or happy to stand up and say that even though we know it is true. Every single clinician in this country, if you speak to them, will know the impact of obesity. What is really interesting is that there are certain lifestyle choices that we feel quite emboldened to criticise such as drug addicts, people who smoke, etc. If one tells a doctor that they smoke, every single doctor will have a kind of soft touch point of okay, we're going to just have a brief discussion around smoking. What could you do to change that? But for somebody who is obese, very few doctors will feel comfortable even bringing that subject up, let alone saying that you need to address this. Of course, that may also come under identity politics in a very subtle, perverse, strange way. If we care about the NHS, it's the one thing that we can do is to encourage people to live healthier lives and we should feel emboldened to say so.

I: What do you see as the future of the NHS?

MP: Probably being very realistic what will happen, certainly in the current atmosphere no politician is ever going to turn around and do anything drastic. Even with the Conservative government, people start saying that they are destroying the NHS. They are not. You know, we've had Tories in power for a decade and more really. If they were going to try and bring it down, they would have succeeded by now. There is no political will whatsoever to bring it down. And really all of these kind of changes, these modifications, are just tweaking round the edges because nobody has got any courage to actually broach the subject to say that look, this is fundamentally a system that was great 60 years ago but it has progressed too far and it is not going to work. We need to change the models of this. However, I suspect that what will end up happening is that we will see this kind of slow erosion again and again and there will just come a tipping point. I have been really surprised by people, for example, who started seeing private doctors online and so on because they just can't get through to their NHS for things like sore throats, dermatology appointments and even psychiatrists, even if it's just a one-off assessment. I think that will happen more and more and more until we reach a tipping point. And the NHS naturally ends in some way. I think we will always have things like cancer services a bit similar to many other countries, fundamental things like A&E, maternity services and so on. So the basics will be dealt with by the State, but for everything else, people will basically pay in one way or another. And I personally find that would be an absolute tragedy. I'd be really upset. The main way I feel of changing behaviour and to try and stop this happening is to introduce an NHS tax. We already have that with national insurance contributions, but everyone has forgotten about that because it has been subsumed within just general taxation. I would be quite keen and I've written quite a lot about it for having a specific tax that everybody knows that it is guaranteed and enshrined in law that every single penny of that goes into the NHS. The government is not allowed to rob it in any way or take anything away. It is just that money to pay for the NHS. Also because people would be quite surprised at how relatively little really they have to pay. They will be quite pleased about that actually. But also it sets up a very easy conversation with the politicians, because although they are in-charge they are not able to deliver healthcare. Thus, the politicians can have a very straightforward conversation – or relatively more straightforward conversation – with the general public about what things they want to pay for and not to pay for. So if you sit there and say, right, IVF is going to be very tough on the NHS, and it is going to cost everyone £2.50 a year. I think most people would say yes to that and politicians can say that the package has been sorted and as a nation we have decided that this is essential. So it stops this kind of endless debate that goes on about what we are going to cut, what we can't cut, what we should fund, what we shouldn't fund. It can be put to the people in a much more straightforward way. A bit like now they have started doing it in the nudge unit. When you now pay your tax, you get a bill back and it states that 20% of it is towards policing 15% went towards this so that literally you can see where your tax goes. I want it very clearly so that when there is a rise in NHS tax, you should be able to look at where the rise is coming from. I think it would help. It will remind people of the fact that this is not free. It is free at the point of access. That does not mean you're not paying for it.

I: I have talked to politicians that all you need to do is have a pie chart and say this pie chart represents £1 that goes into the NHS. Of this say £0.40 goes to staff costs, £0.10 to beds, £0.02 towards ambulance service etc. so that people know where their money is going. But the politicians are really scared of doing that.

MP: I know. I have written about this so many times. I don't understand why they don't get it. To me, it seems incredibly easy. Also,
if you were to be fining people in some way they will understand
that there is a defined pot of money that they are specifically putting in and when they access the NHS, they're taking money out
again. And when people misuse the NHS, they are taking money
out and it might help reset the contract that we're having with the
NHS and society. I think we've got to try something. It might not
work, but this current situation isn't working either. So I'd rather
at least try something. If it does not work then at least we would
have tried.

I: You touched upon workforce issues. Do you have any thoughts
about that? How do we train the next generation of health professionals? Should it be across disciplines, or should we stick to the
model that we have?

And is there a way of linking public health, physical health, social care and somehow bringing them all together? The NHS has
introduced integrated care systems. I'm not sure how they will work
out? Of course, it is early days yet, but I think it's just rearranging
the chairs.

MP: I think this is really the problem. There is a lot of moving around.
There are a lot of managers sitting in their air-conditioned offices
with their pie charts, who spend a long time moving bits of the
service around. But the reality remains that they have only a fixed
amount of resources and fixed number of people who can deliver
services in the face of a certain amount of demand which keeps increasing. And one can call it different things. You can do a rebrand-
ing exercise. You can move patients around. It is like generals on a
battlefield moving soldiers around but not actually increasing the
number of soldiers or improving the weapons they have. I have been
through so many as I am sure you have, different reconfigurations
of services for mental healthcare delivery from community mental
health teams to specialist teams. Of course, we can have primary
care-based physicians and integrated teams. But the reality is that it
is still the same patient and it's still the same staff. It is still the same
person with schizophrenia, for example, who still needs someone
who understands them and forms a really good relationship with
them. It is really quite that straightforward. I think that the bureau-
crats and apparatchiks find that quite overwhelming. My criticism
of the NHS is that a lot of people are involved in merely harvesting
data but that does not really get used to improve deliverable patient
care. Interestingly, we talk about German efficiency, but actually
studies done in German healthcare show that it is relatively inefficient because of the bureaucracy. If you go privately, you realise

that you are following around carrying letters with a considerable amount of repeated form- filling. By and large, the NHS is quite good at avoiding this. Yet I still think there are a lot of bureaucratic layers which we could just get rid of. One of the things we saw in Covid was all these people vanished almost overnight and literally not a thing happened. I remember a manager at work once was on sick leave for a year and nobody knew. And I sat there thinking that if they are off sick for a year and I did not know then there is not likely to be much impact of their presence on patient care. It would seem that here are definitely layers in the NHS that I think we could just get rid of. I would also suggest that every clinician who is in a management role must do clinical work at least once a week on the frontline. There should be no more than three levels of management up to the CEO, I think we should just get rid of whole swathes of these people. There is no doubt that they are often incredibly experienced, very, very good clinicians. We should be able to pay them the same salary. Why don't we pay the frontline staff as much as the people that are sitting there filling out forms in an office somewhere with their lattes and pie charts. To me, it doesn't make any sense. If you are a really good nurse, it is seen almost as a professional failing if ten years later you are still seeing patients. If I were in-charge of the NHS, I would have come and cut swathes and swathes of managers saying: "I'm not firing you, I'm just putting you back on the frontline. You're an excellent nurse. You're an excellent physiotherapist or a psychologist". They're back on the frontline and we would be 10–20% extra staff overnight. We would reduce bureaucracy and time clinicians spend away from patient care. There would not be never ending emails that have absolutely no function whatsoever apart from just reinforcing the fact they need a job and that they are just collecting pointless bits of data which no one else apart from other data collectors ever get to see.

I: I am with you. We have touched upon integration but do you have any thoughts about how primary care and secondary care can be integrated, or is that a no -no?

MP: Well, I think, again, it is just another artificial distinction that actually is historical. And in other areas of the world in many settings, there isn't that sort of artificial distinction. I think there's a massive place for generalists. As I was saying earlier, lots of people go and see lots and lots of uber-specialists privately and they are only specialised in one tiny, tiny, incredibly narrow subject. Of course, sometimes I actually need somebody to be a super-specialist but at others I need them to step back and see big patterns here. One of the problems in the NHS in recent years is that everybody got more and more specialised. And I feel that we are beginning to lose the love or the adoration for the generalists and not recognising their importance. One of the strengths of primary care is that they are generalists. They are brilliant at putting things together and trying to see overviews and understand their patients in a much more holistic way. So why do we persist with this two-tier system? Can't we somehow integrate that? I think it is about bringing back general practice from this kind of franchise model and taking it back into the NHS as a way of integrating things.

I: We are looking at primary care and secondary care, but still not including public health or education in there. How do we do that? Can we do it? Can it be integrated with public health being based in the local councils?

MP: Yes. It is strange. It also applies to things like learning disability which tend to sit in local councils as well. All of these things are historical and perhaps quirks of history that have never really been sorted out. I feel that probably part of the answer is that social care needs to be integrated properly into the health service. If I am really honest, I think that is going to be an enormous and complicated job. I think actually politicians, given the current crisis, are trying to deal with it. We now have a Department of Health and Social Care, which is a nod to that and a way really of acknowledging that there needs to be integration. This separation is a quirk of history. It was because Bevan did the NHS act essentially, and then few years later, did the Social Care Act. So they were two pieces of legislation. Originally the Social Care Act was designed to capture those people who wished to stay in hotels by the seaside in their old age because they could not look after themselves like the colonel in Fawlty Towers and make that kind of care available for all. We need to acknowledge that sometimes people need a bit of help and support from the state, and we would provide that through taxation. It was a really lovely idea. It was to convey that we have dealt with people's health and now we're going to deal with their social needs. But really, that wasn't very well thought out. The intention was fantastic, but it was not clear as to when something become health matter and at what point does it need social care? And this is the thing that's we have seen in recent years, as the definition of social care has changed. So 20 years ago, if you had incontinence, it was considered a medical condition. And if you needed help because of your incontinence, that was on the NHS. Over time we just eroded that and now it comes into social care and so now you have to pay a contribution. Again it is a historical anomaly. We need to think of ways of putting that back together again and saying that things are complex and often it is not one or the other but both together.

I: Can you say something about new technologies and delivery of services?

MP: Well, part of me thinks that this is fantastic. It's going to be a way forward. It is a way of helping commissioners of services to communicate quickly and effectively. It is about breaking down barriers so that if people can't necessarily access doctors or that they are geographically isolated, there are ways of integrating care. Also you can get lots of clinicians from all over the country involved in someone's care by phone. It's definitely got advantages. However, anyone who has been in the NHS for more than 10–15 years will recognise all kinds of promises that were made around new technology but did not deliver. We've all heard it before in various other ways. I still get a sense that a lot of time, effort and energy is being ploughed into this with a lot of hope riding on this but they are not really dealing with the fact that it is not going to address the fundamental difficulties that we have with the NHS. I also feel it is discriminatory, particularly older people or poorer people who might have limited access to technology. I think that it is extraordinary that we can all be pushing all of our attention on something that a fair proportion of people will struggle with. It also worries me that often people cannot get to see their GP now without booking online. It is a pity that they're putting all their resources into online bookings and that doesn't work for lots of people. I just feel that given that we are so sensitive about other minorities and sensibilities and it is extraordinary that once again, ageism seems to be the last bastion of acceptable intolerance, and people just have got no time for it. They're not interested.

I: You talked about workforce planning earlier and generalism versus specialism, what is your view on physician associates or assistant physicians or nurse specialists?

MP: I have written about this before. I think what has happened to nursing is very sad. I think the introduction of a degree although welcomed and celebrated by the Royal College of Nursing as a fantastic achievement and acknowledgement as a career and as a profession, they were hoodwinked. It was a con. They haven't got any more recognition. All that's happened is that the nurses now end up with 40 grand worth of debt. They were absolutely had. And if I were a nurse, I would be furious with the Royal College of Nursing for championing this and thinking it was a good idea and not for saying what was going to happen. Now they have taken away the bursaries and are charging fees. The number of applications understandably have plummeted. And my concern is that what will happen with nursing is what's happened in medicine is that now people are buying a degree, they quite rightly consider the degree as having bought a commodity. When you start commodifying a professional qualification, people can then say that the NHS is paying me this amount, whereas I can get a lot more elsewhere so I shall work there instead. As they have not been assisted in their learning they may feel no sense of obligation to society. We are seeing a massive retention crisis among doctors, many of whom are giving up medicine, going into the City or migrating. We will see the same thing happening to nurses. They will wise up that they have bought something for which they are now in debt and that they are entitled to get market value for and that the NHS is not providing that. I am actually furious about this and I think this is part of the problem in nursing numbers in the NHS. It also means that in order to professionally succeed, and be financially rewarded, nurses are going into management. It is a professional failing if you are stuck on a ward wiping someone's bum. And yet that is such an important thing. All that has happened is that nursing profession has just basically taken the place of junior doctors. And we have then had this vacuum created at the bottom of that kind of hierarchy especially among the frontline staff. And I feel that that has just sucked in a whole load of flotsam and jetsam, just random people that are there that are not necessarily qualified. We now get healthcare assistants who may be fantastic but are not being regulated fully and may not have the right qualifications actually delivering intimate, serious frontline care. They may be amazing but some are not necessarily trained at all. There must be standards in training and assessments. We have ward clerks now doing stuff that nurses previously would have done. I feel that ironically this was all billed and sold to us as professionalisation but in reality this is de-professionalisation. We've seen people becoming increasingly specialised, not because they're being valued, but actually because they're cheaper than doctors. Now, the reality is that that is not being valued, but it is being manipulated and cynically used. Some of the nursing specialists I've dealt with are utterly fantastic, but really they would have been fantastic nurses on the wards. And that has been a tragedy. I think it would have been better to encourage those nurses and to help them to move forward and get some medical degree. I am concerned that the cherry picking of certain jobs. Take prescribing, for example, you can describe it as simply writing a prescription. That is not what prescribing is. It is a very complex set of decision making. And again, nurse prescribing was sometimes encouraged not because how fantastic nurses are. It was because they thought how expensive doctors are. But no one will say that. And if you start saying that, the nurses get very upset. But I am not saying that they're not capable of doing it. I'm saying the reason they're being allowed to do it is because those in power think that they are just cheaper. It worries me profoundly because it sets up a precedent that is very worrying within the NHS. Rather than addressing the staffing issues they have, they just simply give some of the jobs that one profession has to another profession who may be slightly less qualified or slightly differently qualified or cheaper. On the one hand, GPs are expensive. There are pharmacists who are good but population is encouraged to use them because they are cheaper but also the focus then becomes on drugs. No doubt that they can be amazing and brilliant, but that's not why they're doing that.

I: There are pressures on developing assistant physicians and physician associates or other grades, it seems that we are following blindly the American model.

MP: Yes. Which, again, is absolutely set up simply around cost. It is not set up around providing evidence-based care. It is set up to provide cheapest healthcare within a capitalist model. What is the cheapest way of delivering this?

I: And lastly, in your clinical practice, have you seen any examples of good practice?

MP: Oh, yeah. All the time. Staff often go beyond the call of duty supporting patients and assuring them that they will sort things out for you such as drop the prescription, medication or whatever is needed. The NHS is kept going on fumes in a way, which are really the energy and the goodwill from the team. And, you know, there certainly is my experience of medicine is that really the operations, the pills, all the other stuff is actually quite small, really. It comes down much more to the kind of care, compassionate interaction that you have with staff. I remember once my mum had lost her sight and she went on to the NHS. I called her that evening and she was really overwhelmed. She said that they were running three hours late but the consultant came out and he apologised and he knelt and actually took her hand. She was really cold. Somebody got her a blanket, they got her lunch, and I said, this is really good, you know, what did they do? She said, Oh, they didn't do anything. I'm still blind! From a medical point of view, the surgeon failed but from my mum's point of view, they succeeded. It was a complete success not because of the medicine, but because of the way that she was treated. The consultant was really apologetic and explained that they wouldn't be able to do anything but my mum wasn't angry at all. It was the fact that the staff cared and were kind that mattered. Doctors can make a huge difference in patients' lives through lots of little things which matter to the patient.

I: Is there anything that you want to say that I haven't covered?

MP: No, not really.

I: Thanks very much, this has been really great. Thank you.

12 Dr Daniel Poulter MP

Dr Dan Poulter is an NHS hospital doctor, working in mental health services in London. He is also a Conservative MP for Central Suffolk and North Ipswich, a constituency he has represented since May 2010. He was government health minister between 2012 and 2015. He helped introduce improvements in delivery of healthcare for veterans, new mothers and families. He was a member of the Climate Change Select Committee and co-chairs APPG on Global Health. He trained in Obstetrics and Gynaecology before going into psychiatry. He has been a strong supporter of Help for Heroes and helps to raise money for St Elizabeth Hospice in Ipswich. He has previously helped to set up medical and lifestyle advice clinics for the homeless and people with alcohol and substance misuse problems.

Interview

I: Thanks very much Dan for making the time. You are in a unique position both as a clinician and as a politician to see what the state of the NHS is at present and also knowing its strengths and weaknesses and what we ought to be doing?

DP: Working in the NHS, my sense, is that it is becoming increasingly under pressure. What I mean is that patient demands are increasing and some of that is driven by higher expectations from patients, which is understandable. Some of it is also driven by the fact that we have an older population who have multiple medical comorbidities. We have 3 million people or more with three or more long-term conditions like diabetes and heart disease and chronic obstructive pulmonary disease (COPD). These are only some of the challenges that the NHS faces and how we look after these individuals. I think this stems from the fact that in the United Kingdom, the system we have is very much built around hospital care and much more focused on responding to acute illness or in the case of people with long-term conditions, acute and chronic deterioration

DOI: 10.4324/9781003382188-12

rather than keeping people well and better supported in their homes and their communities. I think the challenge for the NHS as we go forward is about some of the immediate resource problems. The challenge is also about understanding how we develop a sustainable healthcare system that is much more focused on looking after people in their homes and communities, rather than picking up the pieces when they become very unwell in hospital. This is true for both physical and mental illnesses. One way to address that is by developing better, more productive community services with better coordination and engagement between the NHS and clinicians and patients. This needs to be done in a culturally appropriate way. We know that we have a very diverse population in this country and we know that they have some of the highest rates of many illnesses related to some of the very worst health inequalities. If we want to address those issues, we have to look at the way we deliver care and services as part of that genuine transformation. The services must be much more culturally sensitive and appropriate so that they can meet the needs of different communities. That would be my starting point.

I: As we know, there are rapid advances in medicine with expensive investigations and interventions and with changing patient expectations and demands. Under these circumstances what do you see as strengths and weaknesses of the NHS?

DP: The strengths of the NHS are that when you need emergency care, even under pressure the health service is good at treating and managing people with life-threatening conditions. The system is set up to deal with that more acute phase of care, which is a great positive. As far as the weaknesses go, I would say that the preventative side and follow-up care need strengthening. Those who have received support and treatment in hospital may well need support after discharge which needs building up. On prevention, there needs to be a whole discussion about public health and public health measures and how we tackle major determinants of ill health. I think it might need proactive and more aggressive legislative actions to address those key drivers of poor health. We also need to understand that the bulk of the NHS resources are always directed towards hospitals providing acute care. We have got to think about how we properly resource primary care services as part of that transformation of the NHS. We must also resource community care properly. The current structures may not necessarily be the right ones in going forward. We need to have a more genuine integration between silos that exist in the system. As part of developing services, we must think about how we break down those silos and properly integrate care. This integration has to include determinants and other important factors of health to do with people's social circumstances such as housing and social care. We need to find ways in making sure that those services are more seamless from a patient's perspective. That may release money if there is less duplication and there is a joined up service but then put more money into social care. In developing services we need to look at how these are commissioned and arranged and the focus has to be on a more integrated system that has a single pot of money rather than lots of differently funded organisations. There must be a common goal which is focused on patients. I would suggest this is something which needs to be talked about quite carefully if we are going to transform the delivery of care and understand what the workforce looks like. One of the great weaknesses is the political system. Hence a populist politician is thinking of a four- to five-year election cycle. They must think in terms of long-term planning. We are in a situation where we have workforce shortages across medical and nursing professions varying across the country which must be addressed as a matter of urgency. I think a proper plan for recruitment and retention but also training is very important. So for me it is about recognising that we have great strengths in our system which indeed is very good for emergency care. On the other hand we are not very good at prevention and we must do more public health. We must focus on genuine integration and that means putting the money in the same place, away from all these different silos with their own interests and their own focuses within the healthcare system. And so integration, backing that up with a proper joined up workforce plan is crucial. I think that one of the key things that politicians have to focus on is the workforce whether it is the current government or the next one sees its benefits is a moot point. It reflects some of the short-sightedness of the political cycles.

I: As far as integration is concerned, often concerns are raised that merging physical and mental health services will be detrimental to mental health services that money will be taken for acute rather than psychiatric care. It ought to be possible to bring together social care, mental health, physical health and public health. It seems like a battle actually.

DP: Yes, I think so. One of the problems we face at the moment is different streams of funding. For example, if someone who is becoming frail and needs support rails or other things at home to prevent them falling, the cost of that does not automatically fall to the NHS but to social care. So there isn't necessarily any incentive for social care to have those measures in place, unless they absolutely have to. The fact that these measures may help prevent future falls and pressure on the NHS does not always translate. The threshold for their services eventually is much higher now than it was over a decade ago, which has moved us away from prevention rather than towards prevention. That is bad for the patients and the society. So we need to find a way of integrating budgets and services. At the present time there appears to be no incentive for the local authority because of budgetary pressures. My view remains that we need to not only have people sitting around the same table with a commissioning body, but also having one substantial pot of money, which everyone has ownership over. The focus should be on the whole system. I feel that would drive some of the change that we need to see in terms of better commissioning and delivering more in the community. This will ultimately save the NHS money, but also support the patients when they end up in hospital.

I: Basically you're talking about pre-prevention.

DP: Yes.

I: If you had the power and you were designing the NHS assuming it did not exist, what would you do?

DP: I believe in the NHS a service free at the point of need because it is essential. I see other systems where people have to pay. In those systems, you'll find that health inequalities are much larger and continue to be exacerbated. And we don't want to have a system where your chances of living a longer and disease-free life are dependent upon the amount of riches you have. We don't want that system. We want to have a system that has fewer social inequalities. As we look to the future, I would say we need to maintain that principle. That is not to say that some models that work in other countries where they haven't got a national service are not worth looking at. In California, for example, the Kaiser Permanente has got a vertical model of integrated care, which is that the hospital and community care are joined up with primary care around. That is one of the things that we can look at and see how it can be used in the NHS. Revolution never works. We have got to now look at how we can evolve and transform the NHS. We must have a 20-year plan to get from where we are now to where we need to be. That is how I would approach it because it allows you to plan your workforce needs. It allows you time to think about next steps, commissioning, service design and budgetary arrangements. I don't think we can start again but we can think about getting where we need to be from where we are.

I: You are right in that we do need to look at models elsewhere and see what we can learn from that and how we adapt them. We talked earlier about changing patient expectations. Do you have any thoughts on patient rights versus responsibilities and what do we do about that?

DP: I think it is very difficult. We do want to educate everyone as much as possible about what good health looks like and what is unhealthy. Financial measures such as taxing tobacco or unhealthy food can help to disincentivise people and it has been shown to be effective. We also have to help improve people's general knowledge base. That is not to say that we should have a system where if someone does choose to make bad choices, then we're not going to be there to help them because they developed cancer related to smoking or because of circumstances they develop alcohol dependence that we will exclude them. We have to have a system that still supports people who make bad choices and not discriminate against people because they make those bad choices. It is a much broader issue about patient choice. How we make it work? We don't have the same paternalistic system that we had in the past. We now have a system where we need to co-develop services and care plans with our patients rather than doing to our patients. We do that with our patients and that is good healthcare. That way it is more likely that we'll be successful in helping our patients to manage their conditions better. As far as mental health is concerned, if we can understand when someone is well, what their care looks like and when they become unwell what their care looks like. It is about helping them to plan and work through those issues. And that actually is good for the NHS because it improves compliance with interventions and improves engagement. It is also good for them because you're actually listening to them and putting them at the centre of their own care, which is pretty much where it should be. The interventions should be about helping them to make informed choices.

I: What you're basically saying is that good clinical practice is about working with patients rather than doing things to them will produce better engagement and perhaps better outcomes.

DP: Yes, that's right because you can't predict every circumstance, but if you want to help people to understand what is wrong with them, about their condition, what to do if their condition deteriorates and what is needed if there is a crisis. So you can help empower and support them in times of crises much better. I think we need to be having more of those conversations with our patients. One of the weaknesses of the NHS historically in my view is that we have not always been very good at recognising the impact that cultural elements have on how we deliver care. Diverse communities have diverse cultures and may also have community resources which we need to work with and across and also help strengthen those resources. These communities and groups have faced discrimination and may well have a mistrusting relationship with authorities including police. Because of that care needs to be co-developed with patients and their communities and we must rebuild that trust which means understanding their needs and working with them. In psychiatric practice, we know that black men are more likely to be sectioned and put on community treatment orders. So how do we change that? How do we make things better? We have to develop more culturally appropriate services. That is the key. We also need to address some of the healthcare inequalities in our country.

I: That fits in very neatly with medicine's social contract which is implicit but highlights the expectations healthcare professionals have of the patients and vice versa but also what these two groups of the funders in this case the government. Partly it is about the rights and responsibilities that we were talking about earlier and partly it is about funding. But it is also about introducing innovative investigations and treatments and not carrying on doing things the same old way. How do we work through that contract?

DP: Even if we had a large enough envelope of money there are always going to be decisions about what can be done and what is not feasible. It is about what the health service can or cannot do. I agree with what you said. It is about having a better social contract. It is about recognising that the society and the state or in this case, the health service, have a benevolent role to play in people's lives. And some of that role is about helping people to make the right decisions through information, public health measures and educating the service providers. If I was going to advise the current government or the future governments, I would say that as part of the social contract about the nation's health we need to do much more. For example, we need educational programmes. We may need to make some very difficult decisions by doing more to disincentivize people from making unhealthy choices. I am not saying that people can't make those choices that we may need to make it much less attractive. So people smoke less if prices are high. Similarly we need to look at alcohol pricing which will help reduce the disease burden from alcohol. I think we have to be much stronger and more proactive on these policies. I think that part of the social contract is something that is often not at the forefront as much as it should be. In my lifetime there have been two major public health initiatives which made a lot of difference. Firstly in the 1980s, the AIDS epidemic led to public education and the focus on HIV meant recognising that we needed to do more as a countrywide initiative to raise awareness and to understand the illness more. Second was changes in law stopping thousands of people smoking in offices. That was amazing. I think those kinds of things were very significant and important public health measures in my lifetime and both of these undoubtedly saved many thousands of lives. In the case of smoking thousands were protected from passive smoking. So the governments can do these sorts of public health measures relatively easily compared to 100–150 years ago. Then public health measures were about sanitation, sewerage systems, preventing and managing infections. Nowadays public health primarily is about helping people to make lifestyle choices.

I: In a way what you're describing is applicable in many countries around the world. Another thing that I wanted to pick your brains on is training. We all train in silos and then when we finish training, we are supposed to work in teams and sometimes people struggle. Do you think that there is any mileage in spending some period of training at all levels across disciplines for example training with nurses or other healthcare professionals?

DP: I think that's a really, really good point because there are two things about training. Firstly, everyone is becoming so specialised that we've lost some of the general skills that we need in the health service. You need specialist modules and general skills. Healthcare is only used effectively when it's delivered by a multidisciplinary team of healthcare professionals coming together. It might also include people from outside the health service such as individuals from education or housing. It is their discipline and the broader understanding of how an effective team can deliver for a patient which is important. Of course, the patients must know and understand the roles of different team members and how all that comes together. I think embedding better training in that respect with more multidisciplinary elements will improve patient outcomes.

I: I don't think I have anything else to cover. Is there anything else that you want to add?

DP: No, I don't think so. If you're happy, I hope this does work.

I: Thanks very much, it has been incredibly helpful. Not surprisingly several common themes have emerged in these interviews.

DP: I think most people know what we need to do, but it's having the bravery to do it. That will require a bit of a shake-up of the system. And undoubtedly there will be people who from their own perspective will be unhappy and see disadvantages in any change. As I said earlier, any change has to be evolutionary rather than revolutionary that it's always better. That would be my point of view.

I: I very much like your idea of a 20-year plan for the NHS, no matter which party is in power. If there is an agreement or compact between society and the policymakers everything has to fall in line, whether they do it is short term or long term. If there is a 20-year plan, then it can shake things up in a non-threatening way. Thanks again so very much, really appreciate your time.

13 Rachel Power

Rachel Power has been the CEO of Patients Association since 2017. She has over 20 years' experience of working in health and social care within the voluntary sector. During her tenure, she has overseen a significant period of change, establishing a new senior leadership team and a new three-year strategy to help drive the organisation forward. She is passionate about empowering patients and speaking on their behalf to ensure the patient voice is heard and acted upon.

Interview

I: Thank you so very much for agreeing to be interviewed. Starting from the beginning, what do you see as the state of the NHS at present?

RP: I shall tell you a little bit about the Patients Association first and will come back to the question. Next year the Patients Association will be 60 years old. We were set up by a part-time teacher who felt the patients were not getting enough information around thalidomide or having good, honest conversations about their care and treatment. As we come out of the pandemic, we are finding that we have patients who feel that they have been ignored by the system over the last couple of years. A lot of patients in our patient survey have talked about a National COVID Service rather than a National Health Service. As we speak we are going into possibly one of the worst winters I think that we'll ever see with the staff totally exhausted and demoralised and patients feeling increasingly anxious about what's going to happen with their treatment. At the present time it is not a good moment for the NHS as various strikes are looming and happening-with nurses, junior doctors, ambulance staff, other health workers going on strike or planning to walk out. Patients tell us that once they get to their healthcare professional, the relationship is really good with a great degree of trust. It is everything around it at the moment that is causing chaos, such as a

DOI: 10.4324/9781003382188-13

lack of communication as well as partnership working. We need to have an open and honest conversation about the health and care.

I: Society has changed dramatically in the last 75 years, but it feels as if parts of healthcare are stuck in 1948 with somewhat paternalistic attitudes although the healthcare is much more technology based. How do we bring those together and how do you see that?

RP: At the beginning of the pandemic, we started to look at our strategy. We did a lot of scenario planning about where the NHS might be post-pandemic. It is clear that the NHS is underfunded at the moment. We believe that for patients to have access to the help and care that they need to live their life well, the service does need to be designed with patients to deliver appropriate healthcare. It needs an an equal partnership but for that to happen, healthcare professionals have to feel able to hand the power to patients. That means that when an individual goes into surgery the first question the healthcare professional should ask is what matters to the individual. At the beginning of the pandemic, we saw an amazing transformation of the NHS but it was all done to patients. We have to get to a place where if any transformation is needed it will be done in partnership with patients. At the beginning of the pandemic, because it was something new, it was probably right as we had not been here before. However, what is happening now is that we are still looking at re-developing services on what the system experienced rather than bringing patients in to design in partnership. Look at the digital transformation that they talk about; it worked for most patients but not all. It was clear that one size does not fit all. So if patients can get into that decision-making arena at the very beginning of the service design and development that helps make services more accessible. In addition, some people are in the middle of the cost of living crisis as well. Not everyone has Wi-Fi at home and not everyone can afford it. And that may get worse for lots of patients who may not be able to afford Wi-Fi. In addition people may not have a safe place or a quiet place or private place for online consultation. So we just need to go to the patient and look at them beyond their condition or disease and work out what is going to work best for them. We did a survey with healthcare professionals recently about joint decision-making, and they talked about barriers which included lack of time and technology which did not allow them to access information from other sources and systems issues. I believe that if you get the relationship with patients right, shared decision-making will follow because the healthcare professional is listening to the patients and I believe that will also make the system safer because patients and professionals are working together. I think that shared decision-making and patient partnership are the two areas that we really need as we look at the future of the NHS.

I: That fits neatly with the notions of medicine's social contract. The mutual expectations between medicine and patients on the one hand and the government on the other means that each party needs to listen to the others to make sense. Because the social contract is implicit, it raises a lot of challenges and expectations which cannot be met. Every two years or so, the politicians set out to reform the NHS. By the time we get used to one set of reforms another one comes along and not only the patients but also the physicians get bewildered. What is needed is a type of map for patients and physicians so that they know how to get to Place A in the system.

RP: I think that is the core problem. In our regular meetings with the government we ask them for a health and wellbeing strategy for the nation so that there is equity of health outcomes. A big part of that is to do with the creation of healthy and sustainable places in communities and assuring a healthy standard of living for us all. We know that poverty contributes to illnesses and that puts pressure on the NHS. These factors are crucial even before you need the NHS. We illustrated recently a a case where an individual had to take out a mortgage to get treated privately so that he could go on working. Now, that's not a choice but a necessity. Otherwise there will be no income and the family will go on benefits. If we want a healthier nation, we should be investing in public health. Linking health with economy, housing, schooling and education, etc. is essential and gives a more holistic purpose in developing and maintaining health and creating healthy communities. A compassionate society looks after our vulnerable and that is across government departments. That is where I talk about power a lot of time. When the patient reaches healthcare often they don't have the power. We have to look at how we give people the power to look after themselves as well.

I: What do you see as the strengths of the NHS?

RP: People still love the NHS and access is free at point of entry for all and it is full of deeply compassionate people. You can see how people worked through the pandemic. The fact that this is our National Health Service is one of its biggest strengths. It has amazing people working within it. We do value it but also we have to protect it.

I: There are several challenges with population getting older, living with multiple complex conditions, expensive investigations, expensive interventions, increasing demands and as you say increasing pressure so how do we educate policymakers to ensure suitable funding is available?

RP: There is enough analysis and information from good sources for politicians to realise that the NHS has been underfunded for 12 years. We don't have a fully funded workforce strategy looking at retention or recruitment We have social care under tremendous pressure for a number of years. So the question is: is it fit for purpose? You can't make that judgement without getting it funded properly. You have to get it to a level playing ground. At the moment we have medically well people who cannot get out of hospitals because we don't have sufficient social care. We are facing winter crisis in the NHS. If I were Prime Minister, I would get social care working, with staff being paid adequately so that recruitment goes up. One month's induction and by January we could have the start of the social care staff. We hear in the media all the time about ambulance delays but we also have to look at the back door as well. It has to be funded properly. It has to have a workforce strategy that's fully funded and has to look to the future. We need to agree on the shape of the NHS in the next five years and beyond. We can agree that we may have so much money now but we may need this in 5 or 10 years' time. We know that no successful organisation or company in the world would ask the question whether the business is fit for purpose when you haven't invested in it.

I: Two themes which have emerged consistently in my conversations have been social care and workforce planning.

RP: Yes, and both have been absent. I think there are three things that we must have: government strategy for mental health and wellbeing, social care and workforce planning. Simon Stevens did have a long-term plan for the NHS which is good but needs a workforce plan to support it.

I: What are your thoughts on integration of public health and health and also that of physical and mental health.

RP: I think the model of the integrated care systems is a good one but it is going to face the same challenges of social care and workforce funding. The integration of health and social care and local councils and the NHS and local voluntary sectors working closer together is a good model. It will help us look after ourselves and our health and then that of the family and the community as a whole.

I: What are your views on joint training of healthcare staff from different disciplines?

RP: In the report on shared decision-making we did was to review the curriculum so that shared decision-making and communication were at the core of any training . An open culture in any institution is critical and learning about communication and shared decision-making at the beginning of the training is incredibly important because it helps cross-departmental working. We have to educate healthcare professionals around how to work with patients properly and had to feel confident to allow patients to have the power that they need.

I: One of the major shifts in the NHS has been the introduction of the targets which are good but they can become a tick box exercise. What are your thoughts?

RP: Obviously targets are important but they have to be meaningful and easily understood by both patients and the system. If you dig deep on patient partnership and design and deliver services accordingly, the patient experience changes. We can measure the design and delivery of your service, then the targets for outcomes can be set. So one of the things that we're looking at is patient experience. And quite often we measure the experience through their interaction with the healthcare service from the systems' perspective. If a patient is asked to rate GP surgery attendance experience then what's done with that information becomes important. We need to look at that to make sure that they're measuring the impact on the patient rather than the impact on the system.

I: You mentioned earlier that if you were Prime Minister you would change certain things. If you were able to redesign the NHS, what would you do?

RP: I would do it in partnership, because that's what we believe. My vision would be to work with patients to let them have access to information and other things that enable them to lead their lives to their best capability. One can only do that by working with people. It would be a service that works in partnership with patients and public. That is where I think integrated care systems are good because they would work locally across fields with multi-disciplinary working in a holistic way.

I: One of the things that really impressed me was that when in the early days of the pandemic, the Prime Minister asked for 250,000 volunteers to help, 750,000 joined up. There is a tremendous amount of community altruistic goodwill. And how do we use that?

RP: For people isolating at home, there was fantastic mutual aid. I think that is why we need community support and work with local communities, so that people could be supported. NHS England should consider their massive retired workforce who might provide support for patients with simple things such as supporting patients on long waits. Patients tell us that it not necessarly the long wait for treatment in some cases but the lack of clear information. they do not necessarily mind waiting as long as they are kept informed. We have got to be truly passionate about that partnership and engage with communities. Another group I would very much like to engage with are young people. We must get young people to realise that they may not necessarily need the NHS right now but that they may at some point so they should get involved with us which will enable us to drive that social change.

I: Do you have any thoughts about how do we deal with the funding issues?

RP: I think the public accepts the fact that we are going to have to pay more for the NHS. It may well be a small amount, but the politicians need to come up with something and stick to it. The health and social care levy did not cause a massive public outcry. But we have got to be absolutely clear about where we're putting our taxes and what we're doing with this money.

I: How do you see the future of the NHS?

RP: We don't know when the next election is likely to be but I think the NHS is going to become a major part of the public concern in that. As you know the NHS has been underfunded for 12 years, it needs funding not only now but also a sustainable model of funding. We cannot keep going back and forth. If we work better with patients and have a learning culture from its mistakes, the NHS will be successful in the future. I think it is going to have a really tough couple of years as we come out of the pandemic. The cost of living crisis is going to have a major impact on the staff. Within the workforce strategy, we have to have something about retention. We cannot keep losing highly skilled stafff. There are some key questions for the NHS and for the government to ask themselves too, to make sure that we build back better and we do so with patients at the heart of it

I: Thanks very much.

14 Lucy Watson

Lucy Watson was previously an experienced NHS Director at board level leading on quality, patient safety and governance. She worked as a nurse commissioner driving improvements in the delivery of high-quality care for patients including improvements in complaints management, learning from complaints and involving patients as active partners in their care. She champions the voice of patients to drive change at national and local levels for better patient experience and continues to focus on involving patients in their healthcare. She is currently working as an independent healthcare advisor for quality and safety and safeguarding, and was previously Chair of the Patients Association. She is passionate about listening to and learning from patient and carer experience to improve the quality and safety of health and social care.

Interview

I: Thanks very much for agreeing to be interviewed. What do you see the state of the NHS at present and what are its strengths and weaknesses?

LW: I have never known anything like it. It is in an absolute crisis. I can't imagine what it is like to be working in the NHS at the moment in frontline care. The number of vacancies among nurses and doctors particularly are just unheard of. I am just so fearful that the staff will continue to leave. I am certain that nurses are leaving not just because of the hard work but there is simply too much to do and they feel unable to provide care they would like to and are trained to do so. They are rushed off their feet. I am a registered nurse and I went back during the pandemic to help from April to August. In the southwest the numbers were low at that time and I was being used like an ordinary bank nurse. I could still nurse and people were impressed at my communication skills. I could manage complaints and deal with people on the phone. The wards were so busy and people were really poorly. As an older registered nurse who had

DOI: 10.4324/9781003382188-14

worked on a hospital ward for many years I did not feel safe without more induction and support to using all the new equipment and policies and procedures.

I: It is obvious that demands on the NHS have been increasing and the funding has not followed. Also I hadn't realised how expensive nurse training is and as bursaries have been abolished or reduced nurses are graduating with debts of around £40,000.

LW: I think that was the biggest mistake as part of austerity. That was one of George Osborne's decisions to remove the bursary. So when I trained, we were paid to train, we had a salary which was not a lot but it helped. I trained in Sheffield. I did not have a car but I was able to manage even though the salary was not big. The nursing bursary helped people, who had a family or were older to come into nursing. And those individuals were really valuable as nurses because of their life experiences. When I went back, perhaps not surprisingly, the majority of people (patients) in the hospital were elderly and frail and that caring takes time. Even doing a medicine round takes a long time when people are elderly and frail and often they are on a lot of medication.

I: You mentioned workforce but what are the other strengths and weaknesses? So how do we manage that?

LW: I think that the workforce impacts on everything. The demand is so huge, and we have an increasingly elderly population. Even before the pandemic, many people were socially isolated and lonely. During the pandemic people developed significant mental health problems which then impacted on their physical health. Not surprisingly, the demands on mental and physical health services are huge and tragically services still work in silos. That is a big problem particularly so from patients' perspective. Patients often have multiple complex co-morbidities; hence, they can find coordinating all of their care and multiple appointments in multiple places on different dates can create a major set of practical problems. The NHS could do so much better than that. They can also manage elective care waiting lists better. If you are a patient on a waiting list, by and large people understand that they have to wait but they would like to be kept informed, just like when you make a complaint. People don't mind if it takes a long time to investigate a complaint if they get regular updates they are sure to understand. While waiting people want to know meanwhile what is needed and how they can look after themselves and keep as well as possible. If someone is waiting for a hip surgery they would want to know whether they ought to be exercising or resting. This simple advice can help them prepare for surgery and likely to improve the outcomes.

So, simple things and advice can keep them engaged. As a retired nurse, I would be happy to volunteer and spend the morning ringing people on the waiting list and going through this type of information. Bringing retired people back into direct frontline clinical care might suit some people, whereas others can be trained fairly rapidly to provide this clinical administration/patient and family liaison roles.

I: I think that's a great idea actually, keeping people informed and using the social capital that we have. We are not using it very well.

LW: Yes. And patients would really value that. They want to know how to manage and none of it would be difficult to do. This is just one example. If a physiotherapist puts together a plan for somebody waiting for a hip or a knee replacement that could be shared and people like me could help. It would be keeping patients engaged in managing their health and helping them to be responsibile for their personal wellbeing. I think the same applies for mental health. There is a real opportunity for integrated care systems (ICS) to really bring together the resources in communities and to create, for example, community hubs which can be supportive of communities and vulnerable people can talk to others when they're feeling worried, unwell or experiencing relapse. We could really nip some of those problems in the bud. I am sure initiatives like this will help people stay better and get better and be healthier. And the other thing that's often problematic for patients is this complete separation between mental and physical health. There are some services, which following a stroke offer good mental health services to help people come to terms with the disability but this is not universal and certainly not available for many other conditions, such as chronic obstructive pulmonary disease (COPD) or Parkinson's disease. The other day there was a programme with Jeremy Paxman- Putting Up with Parkinson's, and he was going off for ballet classes and dance classes. So there is a lot more that could be available but not everyone can access it. Patients would like to be involved in decisions about their care not simply having medications and it is not to say that medication is not important. And that could replace all or some of the follow-ups with consultants. Things that can keep patients healthy in the community. We do really have to think differently about prevention. The nature of the health needs of the population now is such that we need various things to help people using community activities, networks of people to support those who may be isolated or lonely.

I: You touched upon the existence of silos earlier, so how do we integrate physical and mental health and prevention and public health but also social care and health care?

LW: From my perspective as a nurse, one of the things that has gone wrong is that people have got too specialised in their professions. We value specialism over generalism. I remember meeting an orthopaedic surgeon who only did hand surgery. Of course, it is really good to have a hand surgeon if you need hand surgery but the flip side is that we need generalists too. Would it not be good if he can also do hip replacements when he was not doing hand surgery? Maybe I'm being a bit naive, but there was a report by the Royal College of Physicians some years ago saying that physicians had become too specialised. And what was needed was generalists. For example looking after older adults who need good holistic care so we need to get back to generalist physicians and those are the skills we need. This is something for the professions getting the balance right between specialists and generalists. It is essential to learn from those who do it well, again multidisciplinary teams for older adults with physicians, social workers, nurses, physiotherapists, occupational therapists, etc. can help patients in multiple ways. And then from a professional perspective, I still think that people need more training in health leadership. Working as an independent healthcare advisor I see some trusts really invest in leadership development at all levels and at an MDT level. And that's absolutely crucial because if you start to get that multidisciplinary working at the top then they can support their teams to get it right. One of the big challenges in merging physical and mental health care is that the physical health services will dominate and clinical risk and safety in mental health services may be overlooked. Merged trusts have responsibility and accountability for the mental health services and have the opportunity to move away from silos but this is not always realised. I don't have a clear answer. Liaison psychiatry teams in acute trusts are fantastic in responding swiftly to people with mental illness attending A&E when they are properly resourced.

Physical health of people with serious mental illnesses is often ignored because often staff are not aware and similarly mental health of people with serious physical illnesses is often ignored. There has been training for mental health staff in physical health needs for patients, but there is still a gap. I suspect that this whole business leads to cross-referrals from one team to another. What happened in the COVID pandemic was that people picked up the phone, and they found that they could do things much faster. So, there is something about getting people to talk to each other more and also not being frightened to care outside of their specialism. Again, what was interesting in the pandemic was that with additional training, people were able to take on other roles. Paediatricians worked in adult services and were able to do it. There is something more about this thing about not getting so stuck in a tribal field but listening to patients more. By listening to patients and picking up the telephone works much better.

I: What are your thoughts on patient responsibilities versus rights?

LW: I am going to go slightly further back. In the Patients Association, our strategy is partnership with patients. We firmly believe that if people really get partnership right in the one-to-one clinical discussions and real shared decision-making with really listening to patients and what they want to achieve, then some of the demand for healthcare could be managed easily and better. If you really talk to people about what their options are and what they want to achieve and be able to do, some people might not opt for all the treatments. They may want more conservative options for treatment once they understand potential risks and benefits. We had a shared decision-making session with the Winston Centre and they talked about risk-based decision-making. This means giving people information that helps them understand risks of any interventions. That is really important particularly for people with long-term conditions. The decision they make will depend upon what outcome they want. So if you really start there, you start to get much better outcomes for people. And it is possible that you would not need quite as much intervention necessarily. Having experts by experience on various commissioning bodies can help which will also allow the NHS to communicate better. I think you do need patients involved because there are always difficult decisions and newer medications for cancers and other conditions are always around the corner. The communication with patients concerns us very much at the Patients Association. When you look at the letters and information sent to patients about appointments, the letters are terrible. They don't help people prepare for their appointments. When people go for their individual treatment reviews, they could be given better information both there and then but also sources where people could seek further help from. Therefore giving patients information about their conditions makes them aware and helps them reach the right decisions for their management.

I: How do we integrate public health with healthcare? Public health has been defunded and we know social determinants affect health so how do we bring it all together?

LW: Generally I am not in favour of moving things around for the sake of moving. The solution is to get people to work together. It doesn't matter what organisation you are in if you work together. The problem I think is really what you were asking about before, which I didn't answer about how do we integrate with social care when local authorities are responsible for that. In some areas there is an excellent relationship between the local council and health services, whereas in others there are always battles going on because of different streams of funding. Compared with the councils the NHS is given money although efficiencies always have to be found, whereas the councils as you say are being stripped of funds. Working together in ICS may help as these should help people understand the different organisational cultures, the different organisational accountability so they really can start to work together. Having separate silos does not make sense to patients. For example, one patient gets NHS care at home and their neighbour with similar needs gets it from social care and different levels of financial support. One of the things that ICS can do is to have representation from local councils on their boards. I absolutely agree that just creating another structure doesn't necessarily make it any easier. I do believe that in the end it always comes down to relationships. So in the work that I do, I see where things are working really well and very often that is because they've got really good relationships. From a patient's perspective, as I said, there is often a big gap between health and social care. If you have got several health conditions and you're trying to manage all of that, you need extra support and help in personal care which can be hugely challenging ICSs are supposed to have three main objectives. It is about collaborative care with reduction in health inequalities and creating more integrated, coordinated care for people. They are supposed to be really engaging with patients not only to understand their needs but also feedback so that services are sensitive to their needs. It is early days but have they done so? Have they been listening to the patients who are the experts and who know what is working and what is not? Because when you listen to people some of the improvements that can be made are very different to those identified by professionals. For example, in one area, there was a real drop off in young people with diabetes attending their appointments, and yet they are the most vulnerable as they have to manage their diabetes which can be unstable during adolescence. When they were asked why this is so, they said that they would rather go to the shopping centre or meet their friends than go to hospital for an appointment. So for them the clinics must be youth-friendly easily accessible and less stigmatising where they can just drop in. So more resources are needed or need to be used differently, not just providing everything centrally in NHS buildings or hospitals because this is how it has always been done.

I: That is a very important point in that often the NHS does not create partnerships with community organisations who know the community. We as clinicians need to get out of our comfort zone and reach out and work together. We need to be where patients are. People will use religious places of worship, community centres, libraries, etc. which are far less stigmatising and patients can far easily use these drop-in facilities to get help.

LW: Absolutely, we have seen that done with COVID. When I was a health visitor working in a very deprived estate which was two bus journeys away from the hospital, getting patients to get to the hospital could be a problem. I was helping mums with premature babies who had respiratory problems. They needed to attend outpatients' appointments. I remember saying to the hospital that I could remind the mothers the day before about their appointments. I recall visiting a family to remind them and the new mum said that she had just spent the last 10 pence she had on milk and had no money for the bus. So yes, services need to be where patients are and this has been done in community paediatrics with general practice in some areas. We know that GPs are overwhelmed both due to the pandemic and long waiting lists. While waiting people keep going to the GP because often they cannot get advice from the hospital Then there are people who did not seek help during the pandemic and have become much sicker and need more attention. And then I think there are people who are generally worried and anxious but may not have a physical or serious mental illness butstill need to be advice and help. People in lockdowns and isolation have created huge unmet needs in terms of mental health. For many good social prescribing can help which is much better developed in some areas than in other areas. During my working time, maybe ten years ago, the services in East Somerset had a community coordinator who basically mapped out all the different community groups in existence and directed people to these. If there wasn't a group, they helped get them started. They had a fabulous big new GP health centre with space. Some groups used the space and the café, whereas others used different community spaces in the town. These activities had an impact on hospital admissions reducing them. It is trying to work with patients to see what matters to them and then working with them. Then comes the issue of engaging with the voluntary sector and how people can get support through community groups. Often GPs do not have the time to have an overview of all of that. So we must start to invest in other roles in general practice such as specialist nurses, pharmacists, physician associates and care coordinators, etc. but again that has happened in some areas and not in others. We must use these different skills so GPs' skills can be used appropriately. We have certainly come a long way in terms of patients being more accepting of different roles such as nurse practitioners and not always feeling that they need to see a doctor. Inevitably some people still want to see a doctor if the practice teams became more multidisciplinary. A recent report on medical education from the GMC suggests that the role of physician associates needs further developing and middle-grade doctors need further developing to work in general practice. This could allow more people to be recruited to support GPs, but with limited responsibility and shorter training. As these new roles are developed, we need to see better involvement of patients in the development, both at national and local levels with better communication for patients about these new roles and their responsibilities. Patients can still see doctors but perhaps less frequently as there would be a variety of other roles.

I: Taking that one step further, what are your views on joint training across disciplines such medical students, nursing students, physiotherapists, occupational therapists of getting together right at the beginning of their careers for a period learning things together. We all train in silos and then are expected to work in teams. Do you think if somehow we were to change the initial period of training, would that help?

LW: I think it would. I do think that there needs to be some demystification of different roles amongst professionals. Very often, in the past doctors didn't really know what nurses did. They thought they were just giving people bedpans and bed baths,. Nursing is so crucial to safe patient care because ward nurses are there with patients 24 hours a day. They're dealing with everything that occurs, and they may make mistakes around medicines. But then also it might be the doctor who makes mistakes and I believe that there is so much to understand about different people's worlds and also the pressures that they are under. There is no doubt that doctors are decision-makers and they are trained to do that and carry the responsibility to make the right decisions. If you make those decisions in multidisciplinary teams then that is clearly a stronger decision. And knowing about other disciplines can strengthen the decision-making process. Whether it is cancer, care of older people, mental health or other teams an awareness of the roles and responsibilities of members from other disciplines can help and support each other too. A multidisciplinary team that is working well can reduce risk of mistakes, do comprehensive assessments and share models of good practice.

I: What are your thoughts on medicine's social contract? We expect certain things from patients. Patients expect certain things from us, and both groups expect certain things from the government, and the government expects something from both the patients and medicine as a whole. Do we need such a contract? And how do we make it work?

LW: I think that over the years, patients have moved from being submissive participants in their care to wanting to be active participants. And that comes back to our message around real partnership between patients and doctors and real shared decision making. Patients want to be an active participant, but they might not all have capacity to be an active participant. How do we train doctors and nurses to really work together to reach joint decision making and partnership work with patients? Patients have responsibilities before and after the consultation but they may well need information and support to be provided by members of the multidisciplinary team to assist them to be active participants in their care. Sometimes patients may wish the decisions to be made for them such as at life-threatening events but at other times they want to be active participants. Patients need to know what they need before they come for their appointment so that they can contribute actively in the meeting to make the partnership work. Making joint decision-making work is a two-way process and that dialogue is extremely important.

I: Earlier on you touched upon workforce planning. To my mind NHS workforce planning has not worked and has been abysmal.

LW: Disaster. Complete disaster. People cannot really believe it now but when I qualified there weren't enough jobs for all the nurses. So some of the nurses went on to do bank nursing while waiting for a job vacancy to come up. I wanted to do haematology and work with people with leukaemia but I didn't get that post I got a job in neuro-medicine. I did that for nine months. Then, I got a job in the oncology unit. If you are qualifying now, perhaps you can get a choice of 8–9 places. It is mad – completely mad.

I: If you were redesigning the NHS and had the power to redesign, what would you do?

LW: I think healthcare free at the point of access is still crucial. It is a bit like immunisations. When people don't want immunisations, it's easy to forget what it was like when there were no treatments for infectious illnesses and people became poorly and died. Likewise, it is really easy to forget what it was like when people had to pay for healthcare and they couldn't afford it. You only have to look back at history and see things like the status of the recruits for the Boer War. I believe it was. The recruits were malnourished, small and not tall. That was one of the things that led to public health, medicine and health visitors. Healthcare is so important and so valued. Nowadays, when inequalities are getting worse, health inequalities and their impact on people's health and wellbeing become even more important. Probably I would not have started with the model of general practice as independent contractors, The model of general practice did work very well for a long time. I think there are still real strong things about it, but the doctors are too overwhelmed and not all wanting to work as partners but salaried positions. They do not want that additional responsibility. I would have another look at how that works. Health care has changed enormously since the start of the NHS. I would want to think now about how mental and physical health need to be brought together closer. They could be on the same site as acute care. As I said earlier when you meet people from other specialisms, it does make a difference, doesn't it? Physical health staff can be frightened of the challenges patients with mental health needs can present but it also helps people to know that most psychiatric patients are not dangerous I would create structures which were not in silos. Physical and mental health are such a huge resource that we miss out on both sides when patients are not receiving joined up care. Some psychiatric nurses when called upon during the pandemic felt that they were not able to cope with physical health problems. I would absolutely get rid of any policy that says you discharge people after two non-attendances. They go back to their GPs who refer them back. What lunacy is that? There should be adequate administrative support so that the patient who has missed the appointment can be contacted and reasons for non-attendance explored so that help can be provided if needed.

I: I think that covers it all from my perspective, thanks. Is there anything that you want to add that I haven't covered?

LW: No, I suppose the other bit that I would change about the NHS is starting from the premise that people need to be active partners in their care. And that they are experts about themselves and their lives and what matters to them.

I: Thank you. Really appreciate your time and thoughts.

15 Dr Rajiv Wijesuriya

Dr Rajiv Wijesuriya is a GP in Hackney, East London. He is a Clinical Advisor to the Vaccination Programme at NHS England, a trustee for Medical Aid Films, BMA Charities and the Healthcare workers foundation. He is also a member of the advisory board for Patient Safety Watch. He has a Master's degree in Medical Education and is the Director of Networks for Association for the Study of Medical Education (ASME). He was previously Chair of the Junior Doctors Committee of the British Medical Association between 2016 and 2019.

Interview

I: Thanks very much, Rajiv. It is really very good of you to take time. I am really interested in the status of the NHS and its functioning. You are in the middle of it; from a clinical perspective. What do you think is wrong with it and what needs doing to improve things? This is going to affect your generation more than mine because you are going to be working in it for next few decades and coping with ongoing changes. You were chair of the Junior Doctors Committee of the BMA but the views are your own.

RW: Yes. Let me start at the beginning with some of the questions that you had raised. My view of the NHS at the present moment is that it is under incredible strain recently with the pandemic and unprecedented demand, not just in general practice or in emergency departments or IT use during the height of the pandemic. I think the pressure that has been created by delaying elective care, outpatient appointments and the resulting knock-on impact has placed it under quite considerable strain as well. I think we are only now seeing the significant impact on an NHS that even prior to the pandemic was struggling. This is in two main areas. One is the pressure due to vacancies which is one of its most significant problems now and is set to grow in the future, we simply do not have a workforce to meet the needs of a growing ageing population. And I think that is a really significant problem because we seem to not be prepared to grasp the nettle on that. I am not sure whether we have the data on the extent of the problem and how we address those issues. For example, you know, amendments were made recently to a bill put before the government suggesting that we should plan the workforce properly and look at projections for how many clinicians are needed. There seems to be no commitment to train that number of clinicians. To deny even looking at the data to me feels more than short-sighted. So that's one side of it. The other one really is about resourcing and organisation and the way that we are set up to be able to deliver care. We do that in buildings that were built to deliver healthcare at the time the NHS was founded and when those hospitals were built, not necessarily to deliver that joined up healthcare that we need now. The structures and organisations we have in place were created to deliver a traditional model of healthcare that isn't relevant to our patient populations now. Now more than ever we need to be more and better integrated and collaborative in providing patient-centred care. But how do we ensure continuity at the heart of everything we do in different populations? I think that is a big challenge. Our patients are not homogeneous and their wants and needs are not the same either. We need to think about different generations and populations that have different needs and different social contexts which need to be better understood than they have been before. We are now in a situation which is remarkably different from that of the founding of the NHS. We have a much more international community. We have areas of huge deprivation and actually the way we deliver healthcare in those areas needs to change in order to deliver equity so that we can improve health outcomes. I think we have to deal with health inequalities more broadly and recognise the social determinants of health which need addressing alongside disease prevention or disease treatment. Until we start to unpick those elements as well, we will always be continuing to struggle. My view on the NHS at the current time is that even though we are beginning to recognise the value of those things, we are struggling because we are simply not staffed, resourced or organised in a way that is set to meet the needs of modern patient populations in different climates, different contexts and in different areas. I think that one of the powerful things about the NHS is that it is a truly national healthcare system. I think there is a general willingness to do better and for things to be better. There is a desire to improve things. There is a huge pool of untapped talent and potential within those populations. There are so many young healthcare professionals who come into these organisations and want to change things but the culture does not allow that change and they get frustrated. If only we gave them that opportunity, if we were able to change to a culture which is learning and reflective and listening within teams I am sure we can achieve more change and we could improve the quality of the care that we're providing.

I: I think you raise some very important points of which workforce planning remains a major issue. I'm also quite intrigued by your suggestion that the younger generation has ideas and energy but somehow these are not allowed to develop. What are those ideas and how can we build on those?

RW: Let me give you some examples. When we think about things like quality improvement, new foundation doctors or trainees who are circulating around trusts as part of their training and rotate across hospitals often bring new perspectives from people with fresh eyes having worked in other environments but because they are junior and low in the pecking order their views are often ignored. And I think one of the really frustrating things is often because of the culture in organisations and because of a lack of willingness to fund or support interventions that they might be able to undertake such as learning from other environments. If people in positions of power do not listen to you, it is not surprising that people become frustrated, feel undervalued and disappointed. It is not a surprise that many of those trainees then end up leaving NHS training to work for commercial organisations. And when trusts hire external companies to come and advise them, the same trainees come back and are now paid huge sums. We end up paying an extortionate fee to these organisations for the same talent pool we originally had, and I think that is really frustrating. That is not to say that there isn't huge operational value in some of the staff already in the NHS but the fact remains that we are losing an unacceptable number of young doctors on the one hand and on the other, senior doctors are leaving the service in droves. As we know, we train and assess people and their competencies right through their training but what we fail to do is really cultivate or acknowledge excellence or give people opportunity. I also think that quite often our work environments are similarly stifling because they are so focused on minimum patient outcomes or wait time targets that it is difficult if not impossible to create a culture that is about improving things. Also we have a very litigious culture so that clinicians often feel scapegoated and are terrified and thus not able to have honest conversations or dialogues about errors so that they can prevent those errors happening again. In the pursuit of excellence, we must have the ability to be honest in error, so that organisations can learn, develop and cultivate the people working within those teams.

I: How would you change workforce planning and also engage with the workforce in that sense coming up with innovation? What else would you like to change to bring in the NHS into the 21st century?

RW: Recently I did a video interview with The King's Fund about this. And one of the first things that we must do is to empower staff. For example, why do we not put, you know, a junior doctor, a junior nurse, a porter or a healthcare assistant (HCA) on to trust boards? Why do we not put them in the most senior roles in organisations so that when there are discussions around governance or policy, actually there are people with real-world experience of the impact of these policies and governance who can tell us the impact of these on the ground level. It would also mean that staff feel more able to raise concerns or to have input and development of policy itself and thereafter its implementation. It would also mean that the trust boards are better connected and rooted in the patients but also in the workforce. Same arguments can be made in terms of patient populations and how we engage local communities so that we are able to develop systems within the trusts. When looking at the workforce we need to flatten the hierarchy and put as few barriers as possible between senior leadership and workforce members as we can. How can we ensure direct access to medical directors, clinical directors? How do we create regular checking points where people can raise issues, talk about what's happening to them and the service? How do we ensure that people understand decisions that are being made on their behalf and how these are reached? How can they input into them and raise issues so that when necessary things can be changed? Why do we not make regular debrief mandatory as part of those things? One of the other things that has worried me and frustrated me is the structure of our training, the continual rotation across hospitals which often do not have educational supervisors. Supervisors are people who are asked to assess competence and effectively go through a tick box exercise to make sure minimum standards are met. There is no long-lasting relationship. It's not mentoring or coaching which is what trainees need very often. Tutors are not likely to be interested in your professional development. They should be and also take interest in your professional and personal development. I think we've lost that element which used to be in the firm structure which was not necessarily linked with the duration of attachment. It was about the relationships that trainees had with their trainers or teachers who in turn had an interest in their long-standing career intentions and ambitions, not for the next three months spent in a department or a hospital. I would change that by creating longer term relationships with supervisors. I would make it less about supervision, but more about mentoring and coaching. I would change trust and board structures to involve junior staff, healthcare workers and personnel. Earlier stages, I would be keen to remove barriers between senior leadership and the workforce that they are responsible for, which would create greater transparency about policy but also greater impact. I think it would also mean greater insight into when issues arise within those workforces and before they become a problem. Those are some of the examples of things I would change.

I: What are your views about integration of various services such as mental and physical health, health and social care and public health?

RW: Relationships between physical and mental health, social care and public health are incredibly important but often these are very separate structures. So how we think about integrating them? Why is public health not an integral part of all of the different systems of delivery that we now have? Why is there not greater integration of those teams with services and the way that those services are organised in communities? How can we better integrate wider social determinants as well? I believe that it is quite powerful to have public health colleagues based in local authority settings, but how do we empower them so they have greater influence over local policy decisions that can have such a huge impact on community health. We talked a little about physical and mental health, and I know that you want me to talk about parity of esteem, among other things.

I: I think that parity of esteem is one of those terms that people cannot disagree with but it is meaningless in that it means that you do not have to do anything about it. I know it is part of many Parliamentary Bills and laws but as we know the situation on the ground has not changed very much. My own belief is to focus on equity of funding for services and research, access and clinical outcomes.

RW: You are right and I do think that there are various reasons for that. It is not just about funding and resourcing. We need a national dialogue about how we deal with mental health, mental illnesses and understanding that and dealing with stigma attached to it better than we do. Coming out of the pandemic with increased rates of anxiety, depression, etc., we know that problems are going to increase even further and we must focus on how and where we manage these things. Very often mental illnesses are seen as an afterthought in planning policy and interventions. The number of children waiting for access to beds or access to care is simply terrible. Then we have issues related to delivery of social care. We talked earlier about workforce but workforce in social care is even more important and there are huge gaps particularly in light of Brexit. We need people working in not only care homes but also in the community and they need to be retained with reasonable pay because this is one of the most important areas of care. Social care is integral to the health of people in this country. And yet it is one of our lowest paid workforces. Not surprisingly rates of recruitment and retention are very poor. We are struggling even more given our dependence on international staff to be carers. I don't think that we make these careers as desirable as they should be, given the importance that they have especially as the population is growing older and families are splitting and older individuals who have chronic complex medical conditions both physical and mental may need looking after. Covid has shown us these groups are incredibly vulnerable. Frankly the standard of care that we should be providing for them should be greater, but is far lower than we are providing in secondary or primary care. There is a lot more we need to do.

I: You're absolutely right. The silos in healthcare worry me. Health has to be linked with education, employment, housing, justice, etc. There is a lack of joined up thinking and social and wider geopolitical determinants get ignored. I am sure there are examples of good practice locally, but certainly not at a national level.

RW: That's right. I think it is partly how we think about regional versus our national structures but also organisational cultures and leadership. It is crucial to be flexible and responsive to what's happening locally. I think sometimes we worry too much about the structures in a way that we keep re-creating them multiple times in multiple places, and inevitably it creates a huge level of bureaucracy that doesn't need to exist there. I believe that it is a major source of inefficiency which should and could be dealt with.

I: Okay. How do we convince the powers -that- be that something must be done about it?

RW: I think it depends upon what we mean by powers that be. When I talk to people in a number of organisations, they agree that these issues exist and what we need to do about them. The problem we have is that maybe a political will is not the right term, but political means and political will to change these things. And I think that is what is difficult. It is also very difficult to unpick structures which have been around for a very long time. That is perhaps because we are naturally afraid of change and consequent potential risk both at small and large scales in clinical care. This is really strange because as a healthcare system, we have to be better at accepting and managing risk. I found that to be true in my clinical practice often as well. It is about how we manage risk and what we do to try and make things better. Of course, there is a risk of losing what we've done before but we need to think about it a lot more than we do.

I: In your clinical practice, you would have seen patients who keep coming back and really not listening to you. What do we do about patient rights versus patient responsibilities?

RW: Well, I think this is interesting because a lot is made of the fact that patients are very frustrated with the healthcare system and doctors are very frustrated with elements of the healthcare system. I think the reality is not working for anyone. And the resulting frustration is often pointed at the wrong target and in the wrong direction. Those frustrations really ought to be with the people that make the decisions about how we fund and staff our service. There was an understanding in the past that clinicians will always do what is needed and best for their patients. There was a major trust in that relationship. Over time that has been tarnished or damaged by lack of access to services. The strain placed on the workforce and the difficulties people have with access and resources which are really stretched has reached a point where we cannot cope and patients' needs are not being met.

I: Do you think that there is a serious danger that we're reaching a tipping point where more and more of the NHS are going to be privatised? Although the basic principle might remain the same, an increasing number of services might be delivered by private providers?

RW: Well, we are already seeing increasing numbers of private providers now coming into delivery of healthcare. We saw that when elective lists were being cancelled during the pandemic, private providers came in and that pace is likely to increase given the waiting lists as they are now. The question will be how we manage those things now. Do we simply accept that they have a more permanent and more substantive role in the way healthcare is delivered in this country? Or are we going to start to try and meet the demand that exists and adapt our services and systems to meet those needs?

I: Going on from there, how do you see the future of the NHS?

RW: I find every year organisations and politicians talk about being at crossroads or at a tipping point and things cannot get any worse and they do. From my perspective, I cannot see how we could continue the way we are going on. New ways of thinking and working have to be taken on board so that things change. I think the growing frustration with the NHS is reaching a pretty untenable level. The movement towards collaborative healthcare is an incredibly positive one, but I think we need serious political will. And that in itself is going to represent a functional challenge for the health service. I am afraid that there will be people whose needs won't be met. And I feel that increasingly the quality of health outcomes is likely to fall if we don't find clever ways to try and overcome that.

I: If you were the health minister in the new prime minister's cabinet what would you do?

RW: I would be talking about workforce planning and knowing the scale of the problem. I think it starts with data and being honest about where we are. Without that I don't know how we would get anywhere. I think the next thing I would do is to look at what changes we can make. That can be a trigger for cultural change throughout the organisations, creating capacity both in the short term and in the long term for which we need long-term planning that we are responsible for. I would think about how we can create capacity not just in the short term but in the long term with clear long-term plans. We also do need to look at voluntary organisations, charities and patient groups and involve them in redesigning services that need to be involved in the way that we redesign and retrofit the organisations that deliver services and services that are appropriate.

I: In terms of training do you think there is some mileage in having some common training across disciplines? For example, doctors and nurses, social workers, physiotherapists, occupational therapists, etc. so that everyone knows what others do? It seems to me that by and large we are continuing to do the thing that we've always done over the last 50 years training in silos?

RW: Yes. That seems to be part of the problem in that we cannot just carry on doing what we have always done. And that is as true for training as it is for anything else. Training is not only about numbers but also what roles and responsibilities different disciplines have. So we need to plan and possibly aim for oversupply if ever we are going to meet the demand that continues to grow. We need to rethink what we are doing in terms of regional variations and how we allocate numbers for training and how training can be provided better. We need to think about things that matter such as conditions in which people work and deliver services, their incentives, etc.

I: What are your views on developments like telehealth and physician associates?

RW: I just don't think there is any way that as a healthcare profession, we can say that we are desperately in need of more staff and then say, no, not them. I don't think that's functional. We do need solutions that are quicker to put in place. But we need clear definitions and clear understanding of roles and responsibilities, training and regulation and we must ensure that they are sustainable for the future. They must be part of the future planning and various roles do not undermine each other. In terms of the use of technology, tele-medicine has changed the face of consultations. The pandemic has changed the face of healthcare delivery. Whereas previously we were not using it many clinicians think that we cannot go back to the old ways of doing things. We need to work out how we incorporate technology better into our healthcare system so patients still get that human contact experience, reassurances that many of them need and are seeking. We know that technology does not work homogeneously for patients but I think that there has to be a way of incorporation of technology, because there is no way back to the times when technologies were not used.

I: What are your thoughts on medicine's social contract? Should it happen and if so, how do we do that?

RW: I think it is important but is dependent on both sides having a system that functions for them with the feeling that they can trust one another and both parties continue to strive to get their best in. It is very difficult when the dwindling resource means clinicians are frustrated by not being able to deliver the care they want and patients are frustrated by not getting the access they expect and deserve.

I: Thanks very much, is there anything else that you would like to say that we have not covered?

RW: Don't think so, thanks very much.

16 Conclusions NHS
The Future

The series of interviews have highlighted several common strands but also unusual and unique insight from personal perspectives into looking at the current state of the NHS as well as potential solutions very strongly influenced by individual personal and professional experiences. It is clear that by and large the NHS is held in great affection and individuals want it to thrive and succeed in delivering high-quality healthcare. It is also clear that with changes in demographics of the population it serves and shifting public expectations, it needs to be not only nimble and prepared to change incorporating new investigations and interventions but also evaluate good and not-so-good aspects. A key lesson is that health cannot and should not be seen in isolation and has to be seen linked with education, employment, housing, justice and other subjects. Health and wellbeing are a result of biological, cultural, social, commercial, economic and political factors which occur at international, national, community or local, familial and individual levels.

At its core, NHS is an institution. Institutions are not buildings but structures, processes and people. Their skills, experiences, interactions and processes they function under make an institution work. Therefore, things like institutional memory, policies, strategy are important for appropriate functioning for the institution. For any institution to thrive, it is paramount that it must be funded properly and adequately. However, before we go any further, it is really important to look at institutional memory. As we saw in the introductory chapter, it is clear that the frequency of so-called reforms appears to have increased dramatically in the past three decades. It would appear that these so-called reforms are tinkering at the edges and are not really looking at the broader picture. Some of the so-called 'reforms' have looked at numbers of healthcare professionals but with the increasing use of telehealth and e-health, it ought to be possible to look at skills mix. Again, the tension between the generalists and the specialists picked up by some of the interviewees must be resolved by all professions working together. Broader overview of the population health needs a clear focus and a proper thorough assessment.

DOI: 10.4324/9781003382188-16

In addition, patients, carers and families have to be involved in any planning and development – not in a tokenistic but a true partnership way. For this to work and for service design, development and delivery all stakeholders but especially the policy makers have to understand the social contract and its importance. It is worth reminding us briefly what it means and why it is important so that individuals are clear about the components of social contract as well as individual responsibilities. Several of the interviewees mention the need for a long-term plan acknowledging workforce shortages and changing public expectations. Issues related to generalism versus specialism were highlighted by several interviewees and integration of social and healthcare and primary and secondary care along with mental health and physical health was brought up. Creation of health and public health working within health services appear significant steps forward.

Medicine's Social Contract

The implicit contract between patients and healthcare professionals and mutual expectations is never static. As medicine advances and the society changes and expectations of its members change with that, this contract continues to evolve. However, the important third partner in this contract is the government or the insurance providers or other funders who are responsible for funding healthcare. In the United Kingdom, such a social contract is between the government, healthcare professionals, patients, their carers and families as part of the public. Even when the contract appears static, very often it is not. Inevitably, the contract will be influenced by increasing costs, changing morbidity, longevity, altering attitudes, etc. Such a dialogue in the context of the NHS remains and will continue to be ongoing (for example, see Ham & Alberti 2002, Le Grand 1997, 2003, Salter, 2001, 2003, Smith 2004, Rosen & Dewar 2004, Royal College of Physicians of London 2005, BMA 2019 among many others). The pressures on the NHS are on the rise for a number of reasons which has contributed to an increased sense of disaffection and dissatisfaction with medical profession by the public and patients on the one hand and with the government on the other. As Cruess and Cruess (2011) go on to highlight, some of the dissatisfaction with the NHS appears to be due to multiple medical scandals in the United Kingdom and perceived failure to self-regulate more so among medical practitioners. Very often when things go wrong in a team, the burden of blame falls on the doctor who is often de facto the team leader. The focus on dissatisfaction into doctors has been highlighted a number of times recently (Brennan 2002, Freidson 2001, Irvine 1999, 2003, Smith J 2004, Smith R 2004, Stevens 2001). Various enquiries into medical scandals have cost a tremendous amount of money and time further contributing to a sense of alienation and frustration among the staff, leading to low morale. A major challenge to the functioning of the social contract is presence of dissatisfaction on part of any party. Of course, negotiations do mean that not everyone is going to be satisfied all the time and compromises have to be made. As long as all parties are satisfied with their relationships, the health service will continue to function well. Cruess and Cruess (2011) point out that various terms have been used to describe the relationship: moral contract (due to commitment, service and perhaps altruism; Coulahan 2005, Pellegrino 1990); a covenant (May 1979, Swick 2000, Swick et al. 2006); bargain or implicit bargain (Klein 1983, 1995); compact (Brownlie & Howson 2006, Ham & Alberti 2002); contract (Cruess 1993, Sullivan 2005) or moral contract (Royal College of Physicians of London 2005). Some of the terms are very clear about responsibility whereas others carry with them no emphasis on societal obligation which can be problematic. Thus, it could be seen as largely one way with very little responsibility on one which is often the patients' side.

The implicit component of the society's contract with medicine is to do with expectations that those practising medicine and offering healthcare will be professionals and a key part of being professional is self-regulation. The fundamental nature of such a relationship relies on rights and responsibilities on both sides. Although until now medicine has been offered autonomy in practice with the societal changes and advent of social media, the knowledge base is not as exclusive as it used to be so needs a revisit of the mutual expectations.

The term social contract emerged historically from the relationship between the monarch and their subjects where the latter would pay taxes to the former in exchange for which they would be protected. Gough (1957) among others described the genesis of the social contract. Again such a contract was implicit and carried with it mutual obligations and responsibilities. Starr (1982, p 380) observes that such a contract in the context of medicine changes to "subjecting medical care to the discipline of politics or markets or reorganising its basic institutional structure" which is apposite in the context of the NHS. This is not an explicit or legal contract. Rawls (1999, 2003) advocated a theory of social justice employing the concept based on fairness. There is a clear challenge in maintaining fairness as so many factors begin to play a role in it. The rights, duties and responsibilities in such a contract are mutual. Cruess and Cruess (2011, p 126) raise the issue of legitimate expectations. They suggest that the social contract can be regarded as a 'macro' contract which includes all services required by a population. However, there are 'micro' contracts which apply to individual services. Although social contract related to medicine is roughly similar across cultures, cultural patterns and attitudes to healthcare and help-seeking vary. In many cultures and setting, attitudes towards doctors and therapeutic interactions are more geared towards equal partnerships, whereas in other cultures, doctors in particular are left to make the decisions. However, as Cruess and Cruess (2011, p 127) note, the role of the healer does not differ (widely) across cultures which in itself will play a role in the development and the maintenance of social contract.

As several of the interviewees in this volume have highlighted the rise of (super) specialisation in medicine (although quite right as well as important), the unintended consequences have led to a status-oriented setting, a hierarchy and tribalism. Several observers have noted that the growth of specialisation has led to fragmentation of medicine and the profession's unity (Elliott 1972, Freidson 1970, Krause 1996, Starr 1982, Stevens 1996, 2001). Perhaps the solution is that as in an impressionist painting individual dots can represent various specialties and super-specialties but the professional leadership looks at the bigger picture and conveys that to policymakers and stakeholders. The professional leadership needs to attempt to get rid of tribalism which is difficult but not impossible. The negotiations between the profession and the government in cultures with government-funded systems may have to take place through trade unions. These negotiations have their own ethical dilemmas.

Multiple stakeholders are part of the social contract (Rosen & Dewar 2004). These have to include not only patients, their carers and families but also public on the one hand and all disciplines of health professionals on the other. Society itself is complex and government itself can be seen as part of the society. It is also worth noting that healthcare professionals are also members of the society so have a dual role to play. Whether government in the context of government-funded systems of healthcare should be seen as separate from society is worth exploring further. There are additional external factors which are an integral part of the society but can have major impact on the social contract. These include media, regulators and their regulatory frameworks (which will define and deliver professionalism). However, tragically in many settings rather than being facilitatory these organisations take on a much more punitive role.

It is also worth remembering that in order for such a contract to exist and function, it is imperative that there is a degree of trust between the parties (Pescolido et al. 2000). Equally important is that parties do not make unreasonable demands of each other (Feldman et al. 1998), but how these demands are identified as unreasonable needs thorough discussion because the parties might well differ on what is unreasonable and what is not.

Patient/public expectations of the healthcare professionals:

- Access to competent care
- Affordable care
- Appropriate and accessible service
- Altruism, morality, integrity
- Transparency
- Accountability and trustworthiness
- Source of objective advice
- Promotion of public good

Medicine's expectations of patients:

- Autonomy
- Role in public advice and development of policy
- Shared responsibility
- Appropriate suitable rewards

Government expectations of medicine:

- Competence
- Morality
- Compliance with regulation
- Accountability
- Transparency
- Source of unbiased objective advice
- Promotion of health and values

Medicine's expectations of government:

- Sufficient resources
- Self-regulation
- Offer advice when sought
- Autonomy and professionalism
- Properly funded equitable system
- Role in developing policies

Patient expectations of government:

- Good quality of healthcare
- Accessible, appropriate, equitable services
- Accountability
- Appropriate input into health policy

Government expectations of patients:

- Appropriate use of resources
- Reasonable expectations
- Degree of responsibility of own health

Professional Leadership

Profession must assume responsibility for ensuring autonomy and self-regulation but it has to be done in an open and transparent manner. In addition, professional leadership has to focus on a clear communication and ensuring that services are equitable, accessible as well as accountable. A key advantage of working in a healthcare system like the NHS is its non-competitive nature even though politicians have often attempted to introduce an element of competition. Profession's leaders must think outside the box, use allocated resources appropriately and ensure that these provide value for money. Learning from examples of good practice from other parts of the world and sharing these within the system is important. Leaders also have a clear obligation to provide joined-up leadership and address potential threats and changing healthcare needs of the society in the face of changing societal expectations. The social contract evolves by negotiation (Cruess & Cruess 2011, p 137) and leaders therefore need to be nimble as well as prepared and trained for such a purpose. The negotiations with various stakeholders did take place prior to the establishment of the NHS over a number of years and regular negotiations continue with access to the negotiating table. What is needed, however, is prominent voice of the patients, their informal cavers and public at large. This is about the common good not narrow interests. Social contract needs to be comprehensive and coherent and needs a clear strategic direction. Furthermore, a long-term plan for healthcare is needed for which all political parties are signed up to. There is no doubt that politicians on behalf of the society determine the social contract and patients, public and healthcare professionals have to follow this but engaging key stakeholders at an early stage will enable stability and acceptance. This has to be conducted in the context of transparency. As some of the interviewees highlight the professional leadership is important but occasionally missing. No healthcare system can function without healthcare professionals and leaders of professions have a clear moral obligation to ensure that any health reforms are linked to the professional values of different disciplines. Tele-health and other technological advances need to be used appropriately including proper training and ethical concerns being addressed.

NHS as an Institution

As mentioned earlier, not only that NHS is seen as institution but it is formed of individuals – doctors, nurses, social workers, administrative staff, occupational therapists, pharmacists, physiotherapists, managers, other professionals, support staff and paramedics. Over the past few decades, there have been several additions to this cadre of professionals – nurse specialists, physician associates and paramedics who are trained individuals with specific tasks and specialised skills. Lewis (1969) introduced the concept of common beliefs between two bodies or individuals which fits in neatly with the concepts related to social contract. Lewis proposes that coordination can be only achieved by acting on concordant expectations about each other's actions. This is achieved by putting oneself in the shoes of the other which fits in with various approaches in psychotherapy and developing empathy and understanding through acknowledging and adapting the perspective of the other and simulation of other individual's thoughts. These interactions are crucial in team work as well as social contract.

Institutions carry certain characteristics, roles and rules. These are associated with the function and the purpose of the institution. Any institution also has a clear hierarchy and functions are used to understand institutions and processes along with structures. The notion of function is strictly related to the idea of purpose or goal (Guala 2016). Institutional rules can be conditional. For example, if a person A does x, then person B has to do y and person C must do z in order to deliver the function of the institution. This coordinated functionality is critical in ensuring that institutions function successfully. In any institution, individuals need autonomy to a degree within the context of agreeing to do what is needed and go on to deliver agreed outcomes. Guala (2016) raises the issue that institutions are generally beneficial but that does not mean that they benefit all individuals in the same manner (p 5). Individuals will have different roles and responsibilities, and each institution also regulates behaviours of individuals who are part of the institution and also help run it. In an institution like the NHS, each individual's role and behaviour will be allocated or determined according to their specialism and skills. Furthermore, there will be both formal and informal roles. In the complex institution that is the NHS, individual hospitals, primary care services, community centres each have their own culture which influences functioning as well as interpersonal relationships according to cultures of these mini-institutions. Guala (2016, p 1) notes that a social system maintains its equilibrium when the incentives of the relevant actors contribute to keep it in its current state. If this is applied to the NHS in an institutional format, it makes it clear that in order to keep it functioning and homeostasis, any movement has to be very carefully considered. As Schotter (1981, p 9) defines institutions as regularities in behaviour which are agreed to by all members of society which again reflects the importance of social contract so individuals in and out of the institution are fully aware of roles as well as their responsibilities. Institutions have and carry certain rules which apply to them. Rules are a certain set of particular action that are in some respects similar while a practice rule defines a certain type of actions before they are instantiated in specific cases (Guala 2016, p 58). Rules can be regulative or constitutive. This means that individuals working in the NHS have to abide by regulative rules under the constitutive ones. If the NHS is to survive as an institution, there must be certain rules and coordination.

From the interviews in this volume, certain common themes emerge. At a basic macro level

a   Health cannot and should not be seen in isolation. Geopolitical and social determinants need to be linked with causation of ill-health. All policies must have a health impact assessment. This requires inter-ministerial liaison between housing, social benefits, education, employment, justice, etc. The services must be equitable taking into account specific needs of people with vulnerabilities whether these are related to age, disability, gender, sexual orientation, religion, etc.

b   There needs to be an arm's length body (like the Bank of England) which runs the NHS. Individuals must be appointed independently to serve on the Board with specific responsibilities. This will help create a sense of purpose and daily control by ministers may be minimal with the relevant long-term planning.

c   Patients must have a major role on the Board and policy making. They must be supported in expressing their voice.

d   For services to be appropriate and accessible, these must be based in the communities with ease of access to specialists. The role of general practitioner will have to change from simple gatekeeping to a mixture of specialism and generalism. Services must be community based and community engagement is the key. Furthermore, working across disciplines will allow innovative services.

e   Funding for the NHS to be determined and allocated on a long-term basis. Cross-party consensus is essential to have long-term plan in place which should be reviewed regularly. Having a 10- 20 year plan taking into account changing needs of the society and bearing in mind the social contract will be helpful. This will manage expectations and ensure proper delivery of healthcare. This should be done with cross-party support and commitment.

f   Recruitment and retention is critical in delivering healthcare. Again workforce planning needs to be taken extremely seriously and policymakers must fund these properly. Short-term solutions by re-cruiting people for countries which can ill afford to lose them must not be the norm. There is little point in not paying people properly as people can move around the world more easily than they did few generations ago. It is crucial to emphasise that every professional in the NHS is encouraged and supported in their personal and person-alised professional development.

g   Regulatory systems need to be less rigid and a major degree of autonomy in self-regulation should be allowed. They must be more facilitatory and less punitive.

h   Appropriate facilities for the staff when on duty to have periods and places of relaxation, have access to nutritious food and support to be made available throughout the NHS.

i   There must be proper estimate of beds needed, other resources required along with proper workforce planning which should be long term. Suitable funding is one thing but its proper application is crucial.

j   Roles and responsibilities for patients and healthcare workers need to be made clearer and understood by all parties i.e. patients, health-care professionals and the government.

Training and Professional Development

a   From early years of training, fixed periods of joint learning across specialties and disciplines need to be set up so that team members are aware of each member's roles and responsibilities.

b   As part of individual professional development, continuing education must be in place for all members of staff throughout their career with appropriate coaching and mentoring.

c   Generalists and specialists must work closely together. All generalists should be encouraged to develop specific specialist skills. Resources must be made available to ensure that these skills are kept up. Better coordinated use of telehealth and e-health needs further development.

d   Government policies and resources must be available to prevent burn-out among staff, eliminate bullying and discrimination to improve staff morale.

e   The atmosphere within hospital and other clinical settings should be facilitatory and not punitive. When errors occur, there must be mech-anisms in place to support staff. As noted by some of the interviewees whistle-blowers should not be punished but freedom to speak must be facilitated.

f   Litigious nature of confrontation between those who suffer a loss and those who were looking after the patients must be abolished so that people can learn and thrive. The cost of legal suits in the NHS is massive.

g   Individuals must be valued in their respective roles. Support for staff at all levels must be easily and readily accessible for those who seek it or require it.

Conclusions

There is no doubt that the NHS is a valued part of our society. At 75 years with the structures set up three generations ago, the time has come to be bold and look ahead with possible solutions not tinkering at the edges. Practice of medicine has changed as have patient expectations. It is essential that we be innovative in re-designing services so that people who need them will be proud to use them. NHS needs and deserves a long-term plan with cross-party consensus and ring-fenced funding ensuring that resources are adequate. Health cannot and should not be seen in a silo and there must be an inter-connectedness with education, housing, employment, justice, etc. Vulnerable individuals must be supported from early stage. Thinking outside the box working with voluntary organisations, religious and community leaders, teachers and community as a whole will help create health. Public health and health need to be integrated. Social care and health need to come together and health must move out into communities to help them thrive. Models created and working elsewhere must be widely shared and developed. Health is everyone's basic right.

References

BMA (2019): *Medicine's social contract*. London: BMA

Brennan T (2002): Physician's professional responsibility to improve the quality of care. *Acad Med* 77, 973–980.

Brownlie J, & Howson A (2006): Between the demands of truth and government. *Soc Sci Med* 62, 433–443.

Coulahan I (2005): Today's professionalism: engaging the mind but not the heart. *Acad Med* 80, 892–898

Cruess RL (1993): Locke, Rousseau and the modern surgeon. *J Paed Orthop* 13, 108–112

Cruess S, & Cruess RL (2011): Medicine's social contract with society: its nature, evolution and present state. In D Bhugra, A Malik & G Ikkos (eds): *Psychiatry's contract with society: concepts, controversies and consequences*. Oxford: Oxford University Press, pp 123–141

Elliott P (1972): *The sociology of the professions*. London: Macmillan Press

Feldman D, Novak D, & Graceley E (1998): Effects of managed care on physician-patient relationships, quality of care and the ethical practice of medicine. *Arch Int Med* 158, 1626–1633.

Freidson E (1970): *Professional dominance the social structure of medical care*. Chicago, IL: Aldine

Freidson E (2001): *Professionalism: the third logic.* Chicago, IL: University of Chicago Press

Gough JW (1957): *The social contract: a critical study of its development.* Oxford: Clarendon Press

Guala F (2016): *Understanding institutions: the science and philosophy of living together.* Oxford: Princeton University Press

Ham C, & Alberti G (2002): The Medical profession the public and the government *BMJ* 324, 838–842

Irvine D (1999): The performance of doctors: the new professionalism. *Lancet* 353, 1174–1177.

Irvine D (2003): *The doctor's tale: professionalism and public trust.* Abingdon: Radcliffe Medical Press

Klein R (1983): *The politics of the national health service.* Harlow: Longmans

Klein R (1995): *The new politics of the national health service.* 3rd ed. Harlow: Longmans

Krause E (1996): *Death of the guilds, professions, state and the advances of capitalism 1930 to the present.* New Haven, CT: Yale University Press

Le Grand J (1997): Knights, knaves or pawns? Human behaviour and social policy. *J Soc Policy* 26, 149–169

Le Grand J (2003): *Motivation, agency and public policy of knights and knaves, Pawns and Queens.* Oxford: Oxford University Press

Lewis DK (1969): *Convention: a philosophical study.* Cambridge, MA: Harvard University Press

May WF (1979): Code, covenant, contract or philanthropy. *Hastings Center Report* 5, 29–38

Pellegrino E (1990): The medical profession as a moral community *Bull NY Acad Med* 66, 221–232

Pescolido B, Mcleod J, & Alegria M (2000): Confronting the second social contract: the place of medical sociology in research and policy for the twenty-first century In C Bird, P Conrad, & A Fremont (eds): *Handbook of medical sociology.* Upper Saddle River, NJ: Prentice Hall, pp 411–426

Rawls J (1999): *A theory of justice.* Cambridge, MA: Harvard University Press

Rawls J (2003): *Justice as fairness: a restatement.* Cambridge, MA: Harvard University Press

Rosen R & Dewar S (2004): *On being a good doctor redefining medical professionalism for better patient care.* London: Kings Fund

Royal College of Physicians of London (2005): *Doctors in society: medical professionalism in a changing world.* London. RCPL

Salter B (2001): Who rules? The new politics of medical regulation. *Soc Sci Med* 52, 871–883

Salter B (2003): Patients and doctors: reformulating the UK health policy community. *Soc Sci Med* 57, 927–936

Schotter A (1981): *The economic theory of social institutions.* Cambridge: Cambridge University Press

Smith J (2004): *Safeguarding patients: lessons from the past-proposals for the future.* London: The Shipman Enquiry

Smith R (2004): Towards a global social contract. *BMJ* 338, 743.

Starr P (1982): *The social transformation of American medicine.* New York: Basic Books

Stevens R (1996): *Medical practice in modern England: the impact of specialisation and state medicine.* New Haven, CT: Yale University Press

Stevens R* (2001): Public roles for the medical profession in the United States: Beyond theories of decline and fall. *Millbank Quart* 79, 327–353

Sullivan W (2005): *Work and integrity: the crisis and promise of professionalism in North America.* 2nd ed. San Francisco, CA: Jossey-Bass

Swick H (2000): Towards a normative definition of professionalism. *Acad Med* 75, 612–616

Swick H, Bryan C, & Longo L (2006): Beyond the charter: reflections on medical professionalism. *Perspectives Med Bio* 49, 263–275

Index

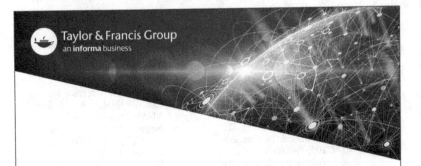

Printed in the United States
by Baker & Taylor Publisher Services